A Guide
to Developing End User
Education Programs
in Medical Libraries

THE HAWORTH INFORMATION PRESS
Medical Librarianship
M. Sandra Wood
Editor

A Guide to Developing End User Education Programs in Medical Libraries edited by Elizabeth Connor

Planning, Renovating, Expanding, and Constructing Library Facilities in Hospitals, Academic Medical Centers, and Health Organizations by Elizabeth Connor

A Guide to Developing End User Education Programs in Medical Libraries

Elizabeth Connor, MLS, AHIP
Editor

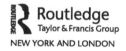
Routledge
Taylor & Francis Group

NEW YORK AND LONDON

First Published by

The Haworth Information Press® and The Haworth Medical Press®, imprints of The Haworth Press, Inc., 10 Alice Street, Binghamton, NY 13904-1580.

Transferred to Digital Printing 2009 by Routledge
270 Madison Ave, New York NY 10016
2 Park Square, Milton Park, Abingdon, Oxon, OX14 4RN

Cover design by Jennifer M. Gaska.

Library of Congress Cataloging-in-Publication Data

A guide to developing end user education programs in medical libraries / Elizabeth Connor, editor.
    p. cm.
Includes bibliographical references and index.
ISBN-13: 978-0-7890-1724-6 (hc. : alk. paper)
ISBN-10: 0-7890-1724-5 (hc. : alk. paper)
ISBN-13: 978-0-7890-1725-3 (pbk. : alk. paper)
ISBN-10: 0-7890-1725-3 (pbk. : alk. paper)
    1. Medical libraries—Reference services. 2. Medical informatics. 3. Medical education.
    [DNLM: 1. Health Personnel—education. 2. Libraries, Medical—organization & administration. 3. Library Services—organization & administration. 4. Medical Informatics—education. W 18 G945 2005] I. Connor, Elizabeth, MLS.

Z675.M4G85 2005
025.1'9661—dc22

2004020216

To Carlos Fernandez,
who is the moon and the stars and Zappa rolled into one

CONTENTS

ABOUT THE EDITOR

Elizabeth Connor is Assistant Professor of Library Science and the liaison to science departments at The Citadel, the Military College of South Carolina. She has held increasingly responsible library leadership positions at major teaching hospitals and academic medical centers in the United States and abroad, and is a distinguished member of the Academy of Health Information Professionals.

Ms. Connor has considerable experience developing and teaching credit and noncredit coursework related to health informatics, medical informatics, evidence-based medicine, and the history of medicine to pre-medical, medical, dental, and health professions students at several medical schools.

Ms. Connor has authored several peer-reviewed articles about teaching medical informatics, using search engines to find women's health information, and chat reference. She has written more than fifty book reviews for *Library Journal, Against the Grain, Bulletin of the Medical Library Association, Journal of the Medical Library Association, Medical Reference Services Quarterly,* and *The Post and Courier.* She is the author of *Internet Guide to Travel Health* which was published by The Haworth Press in 2004.

Over the past ten years, Ms. Connor has delivered more than eighteen paper and poster presentations at international and national library conferences. She has served as the Associate Editor (International) for the *Bulletin of the Medical Library Association,* edited the *From the Literature* column for *Medical Reference Services Quarterly,* and currently manages the book review process for *Medical Reference Services Quarterly.*

Ms. Connor lives in Charleston with her husband, three cats, and two dogs.

CONTRIBUTORS

Van B. Afes, MS, MA, MLS, is Director, New York University Dental Library. Previously, he served as Information Technology Librarian at Univeristy of New England Library; Associate Director for Systems Development & Technical Services at the University of Miami School of Medicine Library; and Archivist Librarian at New York University Medical & Dental Libraries.

Patricia C. Babbitt, PhD, is Associate Professor of Biopharmaceutical Sciences and Pharmaceutical Chemistry at the University of California, San Francisco.

Denise H. Britigan, MA, is Research Associate/Information Services Librarian with the University of Cincinnati Medical Center Library. Formerly, she was Reference and Education Librarian at Hardin Library for the Health Sciences at the University of Iowa in Iowa City.

Jayne M. Campbell, MLS, is Associate Director of Information Services and Education at the Welch Medical Library. She has held a variety of positions at the library since 1982.

Vicki F. Croft, MSLS, AHIP, is Head of the Health Science Library at Washington State University in Pullman, Washington.

Sharon Easterby-Gannett, MLIS, AHIP, is Medical Reference/ Systems Librarian with the Christiana Care Health Systems Medical Libraries in Newark, Delaware.

Christopher Evjy, BS, is Manager of Electronic Services at New York University Dental Library.

Jill E. Foust, MLS, is Reference Librarian and Web Manager with the Health Sciences Library System at the University of Pittsburgh.

Patricia Weiss Friedman, MLIS, is Reference Librarian with the Health Sciences Library System at the University of Pittsburgh, where she provides instruction on literature searching for evidence-based health care and manages a Web-based index of faculty research interests.

Anthony J. Frisby, PhD, is Director of Education Services in the Academic & Instructional Support & Resources Division at Thomas Jefferson University in Philadelphia, Pennsylvania.

Anne K. Gehringer, MA, is Reference & Education Librarian at Hardin Library for the Health Sciences at the University of Iowa in Iowa City. She holds an undergraduate degree in Hearing and Speech Sciences.

Luis J. Gonzalez, MLS, MPA, is Associate Director of the New York University Dental Library. He has served as Reference & Educational Services Librarian at the Mt. Sinai School of Medicine Library and as Access Services Librarian at the Medical Research Library of Brooklyn of the New York State University at Brooklyn, New York.

Meerabai Gosine-Boodoo, MLS, is Technical Services Librarian with the Medical Sciences Library at The University of the West Indies, St. Augustine Campus, Trinidad and Tobago. She has served previously as Librarian and Information Officer at both national and regional organizations.

Rebecca S. Graves, MLS, is Education Services Librarian at the J. Otto Lottes Health Sciences Library at the University of Missouri-Columbia.

Ernesta Greenidge, MLS, is Senior Member of the Academy of Health Information Professionals. She is Head of the Medical Sciences Library at The University of the West Indies, St. Augustine Campus, Trinidad and Tobago. She has worked in various health and medical library settings in Trinidad and Tobago.

Amy L. Gregg, MLIS, is Reference Librarian with the Health Sciences Library System at the University of Pittsburgh.

Gale G. Hannigan, PhD, MLS, MPH, is Professor at the Texas A&M University Medical Sciences Library and Director of Informatics for Medical Education at the Texas A&M HSC College of Medicine in College Station, Texas.

Linda M. Hartman, MLS, AHIP, is Reference Librarian with the University of Pittsburgh's Health Sciences Library System. She is the library liaison to the School of Health and Rehabilitation Sciences.

Ellen M. Justice, MLIS, is Medical Reference Librarian with the Christiana Care Health Systems Medical Libraries in Newark, Delaware.

Daniel G. Kipnis, MSI, is Education Services Librarian in the Academic & Instructional Support & Resources Division at Thomas Jefferson University in Philadelphia, Pennsylvania.

Jennifer McCabe, MLIS, is Health & Human Services Librarian at James Madison University in Harrisonburg, Virginia. She is also an affiliate faculty member with the Institute for Innovation in Health and Human Services at the same university.

Sarah K. McCord, MLIS, is Electronic Resources Librarian at the Health Sciences Library of Washington State University in Pullman, Washington.

David J. Owen, MLS, PhD, is Education Coordinator for the Basic Sciences and Senior Information Consultant at the Library and Center for Knowledge Management of the University of California, San Francisco. He also holds an appointment as Assistant Clinical Professor in the UCSF School of Pharmacy.

Gail L. Persily, MLIS, is Director of Education and Public Services and Associate Director of the Center for Instructional Technology at the Library and Center for Knowledge Management at the University of California, San Francisco. She has worked in various positions at UCSF for the past thirteen years supporting health science curricula through the library's technology and education programs.

Evan Prost, PT, is an instructor with the Physical Therapy Program in the School of Health Professions at the University of Missouri–Columbia.

Keir Reavie, MLIS, is Manager of Education Services in the Library and Center for Knowledge Management, University of California, San Francisco.

Ammon S. Ripple, MLS, is Head of Reference Services with the Health Sciences Library System at the University of Pittsburgh.

Justin Robertson, MLIS, AHIP, is Education Coordinator and Webmaster at the Baugh Biomedical Library at the University of South Alabama, Mobile. Formerly he worked for Georgia Institute of Technology Library and Information Center and the Robert W. Woodruff Health Sciences Library at Emory University.

Mark L. Scheuer, MD, is Associate Professor of Neurology; Director, Epilepsy Monitoring Unit and Epilepsy Clinics; and Director, Residency Training Program with the Department of Neurology at the University of Pittsburgh.

Julia Shaw-Kokot, MSLS, is Education Services Coordinator and Assistant Department Head for User Services at the Health Sciences Library of the University of North Carolina at Chapel Hill. She has worked in both academic and Area Health Education Center libraries. She also holds an undergraduate degree in education and a nursing diploma with experience as an intensive care nurse and manager.

Cynthia L. Sheffield, MLS, MBA, has been with the Welch Medical Library since 1992. Currently, she is Education Librarian, and along with colleagues, provides learning opportunities for the Johns Hopkins Medical Institutions, in a variety of formats, such as classes and lectures, on a wide array of topics.

Yvette Silvey, BS, MPT, is a former instructor with the Physical Therapy Program in the School of Health Professions at the University of Missouri–Columbia.

Kevin H. Souza, MS, is Director of Educational Technology for the University of California, San Francisco School of Medicine.

David C. Stewart, MSLS, is the Associate Director for Public Services at the Wake Forest University School of Medicine in Winston-Salem, North Carolina.

Nancy Tannery, MLS, is Associate Director for Information Services with the Health Sciences Library System at the University of Pittsburgh.

Guillaume Van Moorsel, MLIS, is Assistant Director for Development & Client Relations in the Health Sciences Library and Clinical Assistant Professor of Health Policy & Management at Stony Brook University. Previously, he founded and codirected the Center for Healthcare Informatics Education at the same institution.

Dongming Zhang, MLS, MS, has been with Welch Medical Library, School of Medicine of Johns Hopkins University since 1994. Currently he is Associate Director for Advanced Technologies and Information Systems and a faculty member of Division of Health Science Informatics of School of Medicine. In addition, he has served as Technical Director of Office of Academic Computing of School of Medicine since 2002.

Preface

Health sciences librarians often seek knowledge of best practices and innovative approaches to improve the quality of services offered by their institutions. This book is intended for hospital and academic health sciences librarians who develop and teach end user training programs as well as anyone interested in developing or evaluating educational programming, especially library school students.

The case studies featured in this work represent the ideas and approaches of more than fifteen private and public institutions in the United States and the Caribbean, with contributed chapters from health sciences librarians working in teaching hospitals, medical/dental/veterinary schools, and health professions universities in Alabama, California, Delaware, Iowa, Maryland, Missouri, New York, North Carolina, Pennsylvania, Texas, Virginia, Washington, and the West Indies. Each study is written by academic or hospital librarians involved in designing, teaching, and evaluating end user education.

In early March 2003, a call for contributors was placed on MEDLIB-L, a mailing list devoted to medical librarianship. The message called for libraries that develop, offer, and evaluate innovative education such as orientation sessions, skills workshops, liaison work, informatics curriculum development, evidence-based medicine instruction, remote user support, and so on, to consider submitting a case study for a new book about end user education. Interested librarians were asked to submit a 250 to 300 word structured abstract describing setting, participants, methods, findings, and conclusions. Librarians selected to participate were sent detailed style instructions and expected to submit first drafts by mid-June 2003.

In the eighteen case studies included in this work, educational approaches include integrating informatics objectives into curricula, developing credit and noncredit coursework, clinical medical librarianship, distance learning, and using new and emerging technologies to improve instruction. Client groups include residents, medical students, pharmacy students, physical therapy students, dental students, veterinary students, and practicing health professionals.

The rise of problem-based learning and evidence-based medicine has provided challenges and opportunities to health sciences librarians. Principles of evidence-based practice can be applied to librarianship.[1-2] Librarians routinely seek literature-based information to plan, implement, and evaluate new services and programs. The field's knowledge base can be improved by sharing and comparing best practices, benchmarking service volumes, and learning more about other institutions. Many libraries use peer data to justify funding, staffing, resources, facilities, and more.

This modest collection of case studies is intended to provide descriptive and practical information about end user training and to serve as a framework for sharing ideas on other topics of interest to health sciences librarians.

The cases in this book follow a format similar to the structured abstract, including introduction, setting, educational approaches, evaluation methods, future plans, conclusion, and notes. Some case studies are illustrated with figures and tables, and may be supplemented by material in appendices. Space does not allow inclusion of every handout or survey instrument used by the individual contributors. Readers are welcome to explore the Web sites featured in this work to find more detailed information about a specific class, program, or teaching philosophy.

This compilation includes a wealth of ideas, insights, and approaches that can be used, adapted, or expanded by other libraries. Learn from the experiences of others to form partnerships, introduce new classes, and/or modify existing educational programs at your institution.

NOTES

1. Eldredge, Jonathan D. "Evidence-Based Librarianship: An Overview." *Bulletin of the Medical Library Association* 88(October 2000):289-302.

2. Marshall, Joanne Gard. "Influencing Our Professional Practice by Putting Our Knowledge to Work." *Information Outlook* 7(January 2003):40-44.

Introduction

The introduction of end user searching in the 1980s resulted in "disintermediation, or [the removal] of expert mediators from the information seeking process . . . [redirecting] librarians toward educating users and improving access to information."[1]

Curricular changes in the health professions and growing acceptance of the Internet as a tool for daily living have contributed to a climate of change and opportunity for health sciences libraries. Librarians serve on curriculum committees, participate in curriculum planning, develop credit coursework, and contribute to the overall success of student-centered learning.[2]

After the Association of American Medical Colleges released its Medical School Objectives Project <http://www.aamc.org/meded/msop/start.htm> in 1998, many academic health sciences librarians integrated these objectives into their institutional plans. Librarians realized the importance of introducing informatics instruction earlier than the third or fourth year of medical school, and that active and contextual learning was more meaningful and enduring than passive learning.

From 1999 to 2001, the Outcome Project of the Accreditation Council on Graduate Medical Education issued general competencies for medical residents <http://www.acgme.org/outcome/comp/comp FULL.asp> related to practice-based learning. Expectations include locating, appraising, and evaluating evidence to improve patient care. Future challenges for librarians include determining whether prior interventions with medical students have resulted in effective informatics skills demonstrated by medical residents, and whether remediation or reinforcement is needed.

Over time, end user education has evolved beyond orientation sessions and search skills workshops to include liaison work, curriculum development, evidence-based medicine instruction, support for remote users, and more.

In this era of flat budgets, users sometimes satisfied with non-authoritative results, and user expectations of 24/7 library services, it is more important than ever for librarians to remain congruent with institutional goals and objectives; observe and understand end user behavior; emphasize learning rather than teaching;[3] use evaluation methods to gauge effectiveness of educational offerings; and explore the use of new and emerging technologies to improve point-of-use instruction.

Virtual reference software can provide glimpses into real-time patron interactions with resources.[4-5] The individual reluctant to interrupt his or her computing session to contact reference desk personnel may request virtual reference assistance, especially if the interaction includes co-browsing. Harvard College Library's Roving Librarian pilot project takes a wireless laptop "into non-academic spaces where students spend time."[6]

According to Schwarzwalder, "[rather] than an explosion in information, we have had an explosion in access,"[7] suggesting the use of dynamic user profiles to match needed information to users rather than a series of "boring" bibliographic instruction sessions.

Despite expectations that new services will replace the old, invariably, new approaches augment rather than replace.[8] Younger generations of users expect on-demand access.[9] Today's teenagers typically engage in "multiple, simultaneous activities such as doing homework, checking e-mail, talking on the telephone, and sending instant messages at the same time."[5] These behaviors and habits have implications for future systems and services design, including convergence of two-way communication devices such as the telephone and computer with television, and expansion of wireless and broadband networking. Understanding the nature of "continuous partial attention"[10] may result in better educational design for future library faculty/staff and users.

The following case studies showcase end user education programs developed by public and private medical libraries in the United States and the Caribbean. Each case study is written by an academic or hospital librarian involved in designing and teaching end users and is intended to enlighten, inspire, motivate, and be useful for learning about the behaviors and practices of end users and librarians alike.

NOTES

1. Blansit, Bryant Douglas and Connor, Elizabeth. "Making Sense of the Electronic Resource Marketplace: Trends in Health-Related Electronic Resources." *Bulletin of the Medical Library Association* 87(July 1999):243-250.

2. Connor, Elizabeth. "Using Clinical Vignette Assignments to Teach Medical Informatics." *Medical Reference Services Quarterly* 22(Winter, 2003):31-45.

3. Middleton, Cheryl. "Evolution of Peer Evaluation of Library Instruction at Oregon State University Libraries." *Portal: Libraries and the Academy* 2.1(2002): 69-78.

4. Johnston, Patricia E. "Digital Reference As an Instructional Tool: Just in Time and Just Enough." *Searcher* 11(2003):31-34.

5. Connor, Elizabeth. "Real-Time Reference: The Use of Chat Technology to Improve Point of Need Assistance." *Medical Reference Services Quarterly* 21(Winter 2002):1-14.

6. "Reference on the Road: A Roving Librarian in Loker Commons Brings Library Services to Students." Available: <http://hcl.harvard.edu/news/stories/libinloker.html>.

7. Schwarzwalder, Robert. "The Death of the End-User." *Econtent* 23(August/September 2000):73-75.

8. Troll, Denise A. "How and Why Libraries Are Changing: What We Know and What We Need to Know." *Portal: Libraries and the Academy* 2.1(2002):99-123.

9. "Study: GenY Is Key to Convergence." *Advertising Age* 74(April 28, 2003):61.

10. Stone, Linda. "Continuous Partial Attention." Available: <http://www.continuous_partial_attention.blogspot.com/>.

SUGGESTED READINGS

Brown, Janis F. and Hannigan, Gale G. *Informatics in Health Sciences Curricula.* MLA DockKit#11. Chicago: Medical Library Association, 1999.

Farber, Miriam and Shoham, Snunith. "Users, End-Users, and End-User Searchers of Online Information: A Historical Overview." *Online Information Review* 26(2002):92-100.

Ford, Nigel, Wilson, Thomas D., and Foster, Allen. "Information Seeking and Mediated Searching. Part 4: Cognitive Styles in Information Seeking." *Journal of the American Society for Information Sciences and Technology* 53(July 2002):728-735.

Hersh, William R. *Information Retrieval: A Health and Biomedical Perspective.* New York: Springer-Verlag, 2002.

Kuniavsky, Mike. *Observing the User Experience: A Practitioner's Guide for User Research.* St. Louis, MO: Morgan Kaufmann, 2003.

Regenstein, Carrie. *Leadership, Higher Education, and the Information Age: A New Era for Information Technology and Libraries.* New York: Neal-Schuman, 2003.

Ruthven, Ian, Lalmas, Mounia, and van Rijsbergen, Keith. "Incorporating User Search Behavior into Relevance Feedback." *Journal of the American Society for Information Science and Technology* 54(April 2003):529-549.

Spink, Amanda, Wilson, Thomas D., and Ford, Nigel. "Information Seeking and Mediated Searching Study. Part 1: Theoretical Framework and Research Design." *Journal of the American Society for Information Science and Technology* 53(July 2002):695-703.

Spink, Amanda, Wilson, Thomas D., and Ford, Nigel. "Information Seeking and Mediated Searching Study. Part 3: Successive Searching." *Journal of the American Society for Information Science and Technology* 53(July 2002):716-727.

Troll, Denise A. "How and Why Libraries Are Changing: What We Know and What We Need to Know." *Portal: Libraries and the Academy* 2.1(2002):99-123.

Wildemuth, Barbara M. "Effective Methods for Studying Information Seeking and Use." *Journal of the American Society for Information Science and Technology* 53(December 2002):1218-1266.

Wilson, Thomas D., Ford, Nigel, and Ellis, David. "Information Seeking and Mediated Searching. Part 2. Uncertainty and Its Correlates." *Journal of the American Society for Information Science and Technology* 53(July 2002):704-715.

Chapter 1

Computers & Medical Information Elective at Texas A&M University

Gale G. Hannigan

SETTING

Fourth-year medical students at Texas A&M University System Health Science Center College of Medicine must complete forty weeks of curriculum. These include twelve weeks of required courses (a four-week acting internship, a four-week neurology clerkship, a two-week alcohol and drug dependence program course, and two weeks of required didactics called the *Becoming a Clinician* course) and at least twenty-eight weeks of electives. Electives are two- to four-week experiences, ranging from "away rotations" in which students enroll in electives at other medical schools or participate in medical missions to other countries, to on-site opportunities to work in more specialized clinical environments, research, and a miscellany of "special topics."[1] The *Computers & Medical Information* elective (Internal Medicine—Special Topics), first offered in 1992, enrolls approximately half of the students per class each year. The elective evolved from the suggestion of the then dean of student affairs to develop a course that gives students some scheduling flexibility around the time of the required *Becoming a Clinician* course and brings all students back to the clinical campus. His expectation of a large class offered once each year never materialized. Instead, the *Computers & Medical Information* elective is offered all year long, typically with one to three students per two-week block.

Selected resources funded by CATCHUM, National Cancer Institute (Grant #8 R25 CA6518).

All Texas A&M fourth-year medical students and fourth-year medical students from other medical colleges accredited by the Liaison Committee on Medical Education are eligible to enroll in the elective. Instructors include the elective administrator as well as computer specialists, drug information specialists, librarians, physicians, and the College of Medicine Learning Resources Center staff.

EDUCATIONAL APPROACHES

The elective's scope covers broadly the field of medical informatics.[2] Almost anything having to do with computers and medical information may be included. Due to changing technology and resources and the increasing technical and information skills of medical students, course content undergoes yearly review and revision. Since its inception, the elective has consisted of topical modules. Currently, students complete fourteen modules for the one-week version or eighteen modules and a project for the two-week version. Four modules are required: Overview, Essential Computer Skills, Information Ethics, and Databases. New modules are added and some modules are dropped each year based on new technologies, comments of students, and observations about the skill level of students. Summary information about the modules for 2003-2004 is listed in Appendix A.

To illustrate that medical informatics is a multidisciplinary field and to distribute the teaching effort, the elective administrator recruits others to help deliver the course. The original model of instruction for each module was to identify a willing expert who could efficiently introduce students to a system or resource and give them to complete assigned tasks and explore that system or resource. Over time, as student computer skills have increased and systems became more user-friendly, it was apparent that students needed less personal assistance using computer resources. Now, many modules are guided exercises that students complete. The exercises are designed to assist in navigating a resource, as an instructor might do, and to provide evidence of completion of the module. This strategy for delivering the course frees up instructor time and enables students to complete modules according to their own schedule, creating a more self-directed experience.

Evaluating Specialty Web Sites Using a Spreadsheet is an example of a self-directed exercise. Students select three Web sites relevant to their specialty of interest and use a spreadsheet template to indicate adherence to published criteria for evaluating Web content. They determine which Web site meets the most criteria. This module incorporates self-direction, exposure to Web site evaluation criteria, and demonstrated use of Excel. The spreadsheet provides evidence of completion of the module.

The required *Course Overview* is a face-to-face meeting with the elective administrator. It serves as an orientation session to cover logistics, answer student questions, and identify areas of special interest that might not be covered by the listed modules. With prior approval, students may exchange activities of their own choosing for one or two modules. For example, early in the year, many students want to develop an information tool for comparing residency programs, including the standard information (such as call schedule) as well as more personal impressions about both the program and the location. Students have done this using word processing, spreadsheet, or database programs. Sometimes these "special interests" develop into modules, as in the case of the *personal digital assistant* (PDA) module, which evolved from the increasingly popular special topics option. Students who select this module still have considerable latitude. Their goals can include reviving an underutilized PDA, identifying a new or replacement PDA, and locating and adding medical resources to their PDA.

The *Course Overview* session is also an opportunity to review the elective's objectives: (1) to enable students to identify and fill information skills gaps in preparation for their internship year; (2) to expose students to information technologies that will become regular parts of their future practice; and (3) to provide an enjoyable, decompressed experience in using technology. Some modules more directly address these objectives. The *Essential Computer Skills* module requires that students use a scanner and digital camera, e-mail the files as attachments, and create a simple Web page (Objective 1). Using diagnostic-assist software is not yet a common activity in medical practice but probably will be in the future (Objective 2). Each module is designed to take approximately two to three hours to complete, with ample time to explore further (Objective 3).

Some modules require meeting with a content expert. For example, a new *Telemedicine* module consists of students trying out telemedicine equipment and observing a telemedicine consultation, as one is scheduled. An anesthesiologist who was an early user of computers has continued to develop his *Clinical Use of Computers* module over time—from the early days of Internet searching to current PDA use. The *Computer-Based Drug Information* module involves working with one of the hospital's drug information specialists. Students interested in these modules are responsible for scheduling meetings with the designated instructors.

An increasing number of modules are available as Web-based exercises. The course platform is WebCT, a Web-based commercial course management system. On WebCT, students find a syllabus, a copy of the introductory letter that is sent to them the week before they are scheduled to start, a listing of the modules, and Web-based exercises.

Elective content can be a mix of local and universal experiences. For example, a new module *(Working with Images)* combines using Photoshop and PageMaker with the student's own printed and digital photos to create a personal page for the class yearbook. The required *Databases* module includes an exercise in using a county information and referral database to answer questions such as, "Where can I refer a mother for free dental care for her child?" Most students say that they were not aware of the local database before, found it useful, and were surprised to learn that most counties have similar systems.

The learning exercises are custom-made, but most resources used in the elective are commercial products or available Web sites. The *Diagnostic-Assist Software* module first used the program QMR, then Iliad, and most recently DXplain. The *E-Textbooks* module has used Scientific American (SAM-CD), STAT!Ref, MD Consult, and UpToDate. Module topics can be illustrated by any number of resources.

The elective administrator and other instructors try to identify opportunities that combine elective activities with projects that students care about. Students involved in research projects are encouraged to use elective time for in-depth literature searching, data analysis, and organization of information for presentation or publication. Martha's Clinic is a student-run health clinic for indigent patients where there is access to electronic medical records and the Internet. Students who volunteer at Martha's Clinic are expected to complete a project that, if related to technology or information management and with the approval of a clinic board member, can also be counted as a module in the elective.

EVALUATION METHODS

Students must use an Access database table template to record their elective experiences. The database is sent to the student electronically and it may be submitted electronically. The completed table includes student name, module name, date completed, and suggestions for improvement. The exercise worksheets and comments from students and instructors contribute additional documentation. Since the standard clinical evaluation form does not make sense for use in this elective, the elective administrator obtained approval to design a replacement evaluation form (see Appendix B). Grading is essentially pass (completed elective requirements) or not pass (enrolled but did not complete requirements).

Enrollment indicates the elective's popularity. Three hundred and three students completed the *Computers & Medical Information* elective from 1992 to 2003. In recent years, approximately half of the class enrolled in the elective (see Table 1.1). Typically, the roster of students changes during the year, with more people adding the elective than dropping it. *Computers & Medical Information* is designed to give students considerable latitude in pursuing their interests. Most take good advantage of this and report that they learned and had fun. Sample comments include the following:

- "Cool! I think we're going to talk about starting a Web page for the Pediatrics Club." (about Web page development)
- "This is another tool I wish I would have known of earlier." (about diagnostic-assist software)
- "This should also be a required module because it provides access to drug info that I had no idea existed, and which very few physicians know exist. Very valuable tool and user friendly." (about drug information resources)
- "I made an address data sheet using Excel and Access. This was wonderful because I had time to learn how to use Access, which I love." (about the project)
- "Will definitely make my future MEDLINE searches more efficient." (about PubMed)

TABLE 1.1. Elective enrollment, 1992-2004.

Academic year	Total students	One week	Two weeks
1992-1993	4	0	4
1993-1994	8	0	8
1994-1995	10	0	10
1995-1996	17	1	16
1996-1997	20	5	15
1997-1998	11	3	8
1998-1999	33	20	13
1999-2000	49	33	16
2000-2001	28	10	18
2001-2002	47	22	25
2002-2003	41	26	15
2003-2004	35	19	16

Scheduling flexibility is one obvious key to the elective's popularity. No student has ever been denied enrollment and it is the only elective approved by the College of Medicine Curriculum Committee as a one-week offering. The dean of student affairs sometimes recommends the elective when a student encounters scheduling conflicts, which can happen in the fourth year as students are still deciding about their specialties and changing courses and interview dates.

The college also solicits evaluations of electives from the students, but as with the clinical evaluation of students, many of the questions do not apply to the elective. Feedback through this channel indicates student satisfaction with the course.

FUTURE PLANS

Because of the nature of the topic, the elective's content requires continuous revision as information technology and skills change. The trend is to expect students to complete more modules and accomplish more sophisticated tasks. A 1996 article about the elective[3] describes it as a two-week experience during which students must complete ten of fourteen modules; six are required. Currently, students may take either a one- or two-week version and complete fourteen or eighteen modules (out of twenty-six), respectively, including four that are required. Students enrolled in the two-week version also submit a project. Over time, module titles may be similar but the module content changes. An early version of the required *Computers—The Basics* module listed the following activities: review parts of a computer, learn basic commands, create a WordPerfect file, and establish and use an e-mail account. The current *Essential Computing Skills* module has students creating a Web site and using a digital camera. In the future, students will most likely spend more time creating their own information resources, building databases, manipulating images, and analyzing data.

Another trend is for content and skills to move from the fourth-year elective to an earlier time in the curriculum. As an example, for a few years the PowerPoint module was the most popular. At that time, first-year students were required to demonstrate basic PowerPoint skills for an assignment, and an advanced PowerPoint workshop was incorporated into the third-year internal medicine clerkship orientation. PowerPoint is still listed for those who want to consult with an expert, but that option is now rarely pursued.

Students have many opportunities to use the elective experience to influence the core curriculum. For example, elective students typically said they would have liked an introduction to diagnostic-assist software earlier in medical school. Starting in 2003, third-year internal medicine clerkship students used that software to work up a clinicopathological case.

On the other hand, the elective also offers a venue for reinforcing previously taught skills. The *Evidence-Based Medicine* (EBM) module illustrates this. During their third-year internal medicine and family medicine clerkships, students learn how to ask clinical questions and use evidence-based resources to answer these questions. The EBM module has them ask and answer clinical questions using the format introduced in the third year. Continuing to work closely with other faculty and courses increases the likelihood that opportunities such as these will arise.

Methods of course delivery will evolve with technology and other changes in the curriculum. Student needs spur innovation in the course. A student with travel plans first asked if she could complete some modules at a distance. That prompted putting some of the modules on WebCT. Students understand, though, that they cannot be enrolled in the elective and another course or be on vacation at the same time. Students may work on elective modules before or after the scheduled elective, although they must submit their elective database within ten days of scheduled completion.

Although a Web-based curriculum has the advantage of being accessible at any time and from other locations, there may be future interest in modules designed for students working together, which is now permitted but not expected. For example, observation suggests that students working up clinical cases in a group have lively discussions about appropriate diagnoses, tests, and treatment. Students in groups seem to learn in a way that is different from interactions with an instructor and probably different from completing the assignment on their own.

The elective will most likely evolve to have enough Web-based modules to meet course requirements but still include face-to-face learning opportunities and, perhaps, collaborative activities. Not every module belongs on the Web. A mix of face-to-face and Web modules maintains a personal dimension while providing considerable latitude in completing the modules. Even Web-based modules have a person identified as the contact for that module. A Web-based-only elective would not help students realize the interdisciplinary nature of medical information management, and the essential role of physicians in helping to design useful systems.

The involvement of clinicians is particularly valuable because they serve as important role models for most medical students. As more local clinicians use, develop, and evaluate medical information systems, attempts will be made to recruit them as module instructors.

Collaboration and technology make it possible to deliver the course year-round. Students are less dependent on the physical presence of the elective administrator (who is only at the clinical campus two days each week) because other instructors are involved and many modules are Web based. Including others as contacts with defined responsibilities incorporates expertise beyond that of the elective administrator.

Many other specialists enjoy the opportunity to work with medical students and, because not all students select the same modules, the time investment is reasonable. Before exercises were put on the Web, the course administrator spent approximately four to six hours per student providing navigational assistance. That was appropriate in the early 1990s when students had minimal experience with the Internet and medical software. The need for change was apparent when students started "clicking" ahead of the instructor. Now students complete Web-based modules on their own and have access (on-site in the Learning Resources Center or by e-mail) to people who are familiar with the exercises. The next logical step will be to get official approval for students to take the elective off-site, where, with some advanced planning, they could even identify local experts (such as drug information specialists, telemedicine staff, or librarians) to serve as module instructors. The advantage would be that they could extend their stay in a place where they may want to apply for residency and learn more about the information resources at that institution.

CONCLUSION

Change, collaboration, flexibility, and opportunity are the key characteristics of the *Computers & Medical Information* elective. The content and delivery of the course must reflect current resources and methods. This means that sometimes the elective administrator learns along with the students, which is one reason why collaboration with other experts is so important. Students and the administration appreciate the scheduling flexibility; no student has ever been denied enrollment. Although some students end up taking the course primarily because of scheduling, all students who have enrolled have successfully completed the elective and last-minute enrollees tend to be grateful to have solved a scheduling problem with a useful and enjoyable alternative. The elective administrator particularly appreciates the time flexibility afforded by putting much of the curriculum on the Web. It makes it much more feasible to add more modules.

Last, some might argue that most of the topics covered in the *Computers & Medical Information* elective belong in the required curriculum. The author agrees, but there is considerably more opportunity to develop and get approval for an elective, and, as noted earlier, many of the topics previously taught in the elective are now taught earlier in the curriculum and some current modules reinforce previously acquired skills. The fun challenge is staying one step ahead of the students and using current technology and resources to design learning experiences that improve medical students' information management skills.

APPENDIX A: COMPUTERS & MEDICAL INFORMATION ELECTIVE (IMED-989301) 2003-2004 MODULES

Module	Main Objective or Task	Format
Course Overview[a]	Orientation; identify special interests	In-person
Databases[a]	Answer questions using a social services database; learn about and use relational database software	Web
Essential Computer Skills[a]	Demonstrate proficiency in current, basic activities	Web
Information Ethics[a]	Complete copyright quiz; learn about cookies and computer privacy; read about HIPAA	Web
CATCHUM Project	Complete activity related to cancer prevention curriculum	In-person
Clinical Case Simulations	Complete several cases; answer questions	Web
Clinical Use of Computers	Meet with clinician and review current use of systems	In-person
Computer-Based Assessment	Complete and evaluate tests	Web/ CD-ROM
Connectivity Software	Configure home computer for dial-up access	Handout
Consumer Health Information	Explore and compare patient education materials	Web
Data Analysis	Read review of simple data analysis and complete exercises	CD-ROM
Diagnostic-Assist Software	Work up a CPC using software; evaluate performance	Web
Drug Information on Computer	Work with hospital drug information specialist and system	In-person
Electronic Textbooks	Use and evaluate various online textbooks	Web
Evaluating Specialty Web Sites Using a Spreadsheet	Identify and evaluate Web sites using published criteria	Web
Evidence-Based Medicine	Formulate and answer clinical questions	Web

Module	Main Objective or Task	Format
Information Mastery	Complete chapter in tutorial on critically reviewing a journal article	Web
Internet Search Engines	Complete online exercises	Web
Martha's Clinic Computer Resources	Activity related to computer use in clinic	Approval
MS Applications	Work with computer trainers	In-person
MS Access	Complete online tutorial	Web
PDAs	Upgrade/select PDA resources	Approval
Presenting Research	Design poster presenting research	Web
PubMed	Complete tutorial; do searches	Web
Telemedicine	Use telemedicine equipment; observe session	In-person
Working with Images	Create personal page for yearbook	Web
Special Topics		Approval

aRequired module.

APPENDIX B: COMPUTERS & MEDICAL INFORMATION ELECTIVE (IMED-989301) EVALUATION

_____ completed the elective on _____.
The purpose of the elective is to improve students' skills in finding and managing medical information. The standard evaluation form does not fit the nature of this elective; this is used in its place. Several people worked with this student during the elective. This student:

1. Met the content requirements of the elective by completing the following modules:

_____ Course Overview (required)	_____ Essential Computer Skills (required)
_____ Databases (required)	_____ Information Ethics (required)
_____ Analyzing Data—Part 1	_____ Analyzing Data—Part 2
_____ CATCHUM Project	_____ Clinical Case Simulations
_____ Clinical Use of Technology	_____ Computer-Assisted Diagnosis
_____ Computer-Based Assessment	_____ Connectivity Software
_____ Consumer Health Information	_____ Drug Information on Computer
_____ Electronic Textbooks	_____ Evaluating Specialty Web Sites
_____ Evidence-Based Medicine Practice	_____ Information Mastery
_____ Internet Search Engines	_____ Martha's Clinic Computer Resources
_____ MS Access	_____ PDA Applications and Resources
_____ Presenting Research	_____ PubMed
_____ Telemedicine	_____ Working with Images
_____ Special topic _____	

2. Demonstrated independent learning skills, e.g., scheduled own course of study, consulted mentors as needed.
3. Worked effectively and professionally with various information specialists including computer experts, librarians, pharmacists, and physicians.

Other comments:

_____ Course Coordinator _____ Date

NOTES

1. Texas A&M University System, Health Science Center College of Medicine. "Temple Campus Fourth Year Electives." Available: <http://medicine.tamu.edu/elective/main2.html>.

2. Association of American Medical Colleges. "Contemporary Issues in Medicine: Medical Informatics and Population Health." Available: <http://www.aamc.org/meded/msop/start.htm>.

3. Hannigan, Gale G., Bartold, Stephen P., and Browne, Barry A. "Computers and Medical Information: An Elective for Fourth-Year Medical Students." *Medical Reference Services Quarterly* 15(Winter 1996):81-88.

Chapter 2

Instructional Outreach and Liaison to a Veterinary Medicine Program at Washington State University

Sarah K. McCord
Vicki F. Croft

SETTING

The Washington State University (WSU) Health Sciences Library (HSL) is a specialized academic library at a land-grant public university located in Pullman, Washington. The HSL is an important resource for students, faculty, and staff of the College of Veterinary Medicine (CVM), as well as those in other disciplines. The library is part of the WSU Libraries, which collectively hold more than two million volumes, and is one of nine designated Resource Libraries in the five-state National Network of Libraries of Medicine/Pacific Northwest Region (NNLM/PNR). The HSL collections include more than 65,000 volumes, with approximately 700 current journal titles.

The HSL provides extensive support for WSU faculty, staff, and students requiring information on biomedical topics, as well as practicing veterinarians, pharmacists, and physicians. Services range from in-person and e-mail reference assistance to consultation on research projects and specialized library instruction and information literacy sessions. In addition to both print and electronic books and journals, the library also offers course reserves, reference materials, public photocopiers, a public scanner, eighty-eight seats for study space, and twenty public computers for conducting library research. Remote access to medical and veterinary resources is provided whenever possible, and library faculty and staff provide technology assistance to users who do not visit the physical library in person. Many of

15

these activities foster close relationships between the HSL and its patrons. This case study focuses on course planning and liaison work with faculty members, and instruction targeted to graduate and professional students, faculty, and residents in the CVM.

BACKGROUND

Significant research has been done on the information needs of, searching techniques employed by, and instruction targeted to physicians and medical students studying "human medicine."[1-7] Although much of the information in these studies can apply to veterinary students and veterinarians, the unique demands of the profession require some adaptation. For example, veterinarians must tailor their information-seeking behavior not only to the clinical signs and symptoms present in the patient, but also based on the species that presents the problem. The indexing for veterinary-related information in PubMed is not always complete, and a search using common veterinary terms such as "canine" may give unexpected results, such as countless articles on human dentistry ("canine teeth"). With the exception of PubMed[8] and AGRICOLA,[9] the catalog of the National Agricultural Library, the primary indexes to the veterinary literature are not freely available over the Internet. Veterinarians in practice rarely have easy access to hospital libraries and professional librarians, except through services provided by NNLM Resource Libraries, and must rely more heavily on reading personal copies of journal subscriptions and textbooks, networking with colleagues, and using the Internet to gain access to current information.[10-11]

The application of evidence-based practice and subsequent development of evidence-based search strategies for veterinary topics is still in its infancy.[12] Although many veterinary medical students see the library as a place to study, make copies, and access reserve materials, increasing numbers of students value its computerized resources.[13-14]

EDUCATIONAL APPROACHES

HSL librarians have used a variety of methods to foster student learning and strong liaison relationships with CVM faculty and professional students. All students in the Doctor of Veterinary Medicine professional program receive a minimum of three mandatory library instruction sessions. The initial session takes place early in the first professional year, and the second is part of the students' preparation for a problem-based learning intensive called *Diagnostic Challenges* (DCs). In addition, students are provided with an additional brief instruction session when they begin work on their senior paper, a required independent research project that is presented and submitted during their fourth professional year.

In the first two weeks of the first professional year, veterinary medical students attend a mandatory one-hour library orientation and introduction to database searching. A similar orientation is provided to new fourth-year students transferring from non-U.S. veterinary medical schools. Students are given a brief tour of the physical library, which includes a discussion of copying and reserve policies, interlibrary loan services, and general information on such things as library hours and fines for overdue materials. The second part of the orientation includes an introduction to searching the veterinary literature in VETCD,[15] BEASTCD,[16] and PubMed, as well as the basics of using the library catalog and special tools such as SFX context-sensitive reference linking software.[17] The sessions are scheduled with the help of the student services office of the CVM, and typically are taught to between nine and twelve students. The small class size means that librarians teach many classes in a two-week period, but it seems to make the students more comfortable in what can be an unfamiliar environment. Like medical students, these students are smart and competitive, and they are somewhat reluctant to ask questions or show unfamiliarity with material early in the first year. Librarians ensure that the overall tone of the sessions places emphasis on the wide range of resources available remotely, such as databases and electronic journals, as well as on the library as a desirable and comfortable place for student learning, pointing out comfortable chairs and collaborative work spaces, and introducing library staff and temporary employees. Every year, many students remark that they would have benefited from such an orientation at their undergraduate institutions.

Librarians also participate in curricular development for DCs, serve on the Diagnostic Challenges Planning Committee, and support the program. DCs take place three times during the second professional year and are an intensive departure from the typical course schedule. The purposes of the DCs are to decrease discipline-based compartmentalization of the curriculum, increase the opportunities for active learning, develop students' interpersonal and communication skills, and promote independent learning skills.[18] The CVM began the development of the DCs during the early 1990s, hosting a two-day faculty development symposium on problem-based learning. One of the HSL librarians accepted an invitation from the CVM to attend this session, and participated in the earliest stages of the program design. The program has grown from an experimental collaboration between several colleagues who teach in the second professional year into a model of curricular integration that has won several teaching awards.

During each weeklong DC, most regular lecture and lab sessions are canceled. Instead, students are put into teams and immersed in a case situation, usually drawn from the records of the WSU Veterinary Teaching Hospital. Volunteers and visiting clinicians role-play clients, and veterinary faculty members act as case facilitators, giving out information on the animal and its condition in response to questions and clinical decisions made by the student teams. All cases are based on disease states or conditions that have not been explicitly covered in class, and each DC section includes at least one large animal case and one exotic animal case. Students are responsible for ordering diagnostic tests and interpreting lab values; keeping accurate medical records; working through client issues; remaining aware of legal and public health implications; and creating caring, cost-effective treatment plans. At the end of the week, the teams present synopses of their cases and the clinical reasoning processes used to design treatment regimens. A literature search is a required part of these assignments.

Over the years, a variety of strategies have been employed to help students understand why a literature search is important as well as how to complete one. Library support for the DCs has taken many forms, and, like the DCs themselves, is regarded as an evolving process by librarians and veterinary faculty. Early on, the HSL supported the program by purchasing additional copies of heavily used reserve books, and labeling reserve books of particular importance with labels that prohibited removal from the HSL during the DC exercise. Recently, the HSL began a checkout system for a limited number of copy cards purchased by the CVM specifically for use by students participating in DCs. The students are delighted with this most recent addition and have for the most part used the cards in a conservative manner.

Initially, instruction targeted to DC participants was somewhat informal, and the librarians did most of the teaching as part of the reference interview with individual students. Later, as the DC program became more established, a DC Literature Search Web page[19] was created as part of the overall DC Web site.[20] Although the Web page addressed the basics, students were uncertain about applying the search process to a case, as compared to a research paper, and faculty members noticed that many literature searches were not well constructed. With the growth of the World Wide Web, more students were doing searches using Internet search engines and bypassing library resources entirely, and the quality of the case analysis and sources cited fell dramatically.

An hour-long drop-in library instruction session was organized in response to faculty concerns about the selection and appropriate use of electronic sources. Unfortunately, not a single student attended the first instruction session that was offered on an optional basis. Analysis of this situation by the Diagnostic Challenges Planning Committee resulted in several possible explanations, including not enough publicity, not enough verbal encouragement from CVM faculty to attend the class, and, most important, that students had already completed two of three DCs without the class and were less motivated to attend the session scheduled before the last exercise. The following year, optional instruction sessions were attempted again, with some success. Student teams usually delegated one person to attend the session on behalf of the team, and although participation was limited, it was also enthusiastic.

This approach did improve the quality of the literature searches submitted by student teams. However, librarians and veterinary school faculty members were still concerned that not all students were receiving information that would be critical to their success later on, either when they were writing their senior paper, or when they entered professional practice. The Diagnostic Challenges Planning Committee decided to include the library search refresher during a mandatory lab section, in conjunction with an introduction to writing problem-oriented medical records and treatment plans. This session begins with a practicing clinician outlining the SOAP technique for analyzing clinical situations. SOAP stands for Subjective assessments, such as listlessness; Objective clinical results, such as lab values; Assessment, including differential diagnoses; and Plan for treatment.[21] It is applied to every problem that the animal currently presents with.

The librarian builds on the SOAP format introduced by the clinician to show how to develop effective search strategies in VETCD/ BEASTCD and PubMed using the progress notes for the animal. A short brainstorming session using a hypothetical case illustrates how to move from the question at hand to the use of Boolean operators within search statements. Students are encouraged to begin the literature search early in the case and to focus initially on diagnostically useful problems. These are called "high-yield problems," which point to disease in a specific body part or system, rather than "low-yield problems" such as lethargy, which can be caused by problems in many different body parts or systems. The librarian also hands out a summary sheet that recapitulates the main points of the session and provides a list of additional resources (such as legal resources or links to departments of public health) that may be of value in certain cases.

A team that delegated the literature search to a student who did not attend the lab session provided an unexpected control group for this new approach. The group made an incorrect initial diagnosis and did not gain important differential diagnosis and treatment plan information from the current literature, because the search was done after the fact on the morning of the case summary presentation. The students ended up using outdated and inappropriate sources to produce the final report and submitted a literature search that did not use any of the search techniques outlined in the library instruction session. Although the students on this team did suffer the consequences of a significantly lower grade on the project, they also learned the importance of using current research in everyday practice. Two students on this team subsequently asked for personalized database instruction to build their search skills.

Veterinary faculty who grade the DC assignments agree that this session clearly meets the desired goals of delivering library instruction content to a substantial majority of students and maintaining or improving literature search quality. Librarians have noted additional unexpected benefits as well. Students are able to immediately make the connection between practice demands and the need for current information, and having the librarian team teach with a clinician has increased students' perception of the importance of the literature search. In addition, students have reported anecdotally that they are now better able to understand the idea of a controlled subject vocabulary in a database, because the medical record and SOAP use what is, in a sense, a controlled vocabulary of medical or veterinary terms to describe the condition of the animal.

Our experience also supports findings at other institutions, which noted a dramatic increase in library use associated with problem-based learning activities.[14,22] Before the HSL purchased "binding saving" copiers, a number of books and bound journals containing key articles or background information were damaged by heavy use. During one year, CVM faculty made multiple copies of key sources and tucked them into the appropriate book or journal. Students who found these sources would take one copy of the article for their team, leaving the rest for other teams. Fortunately, technological advances in copier design have rendered these measures unnecessary.

Along with extensive involvement with the professional student curriculum, librarians are invited to give periodic resource update seminars to faculty. Orientation and instructional sessions are also provided to residents, interns, and house officers at the Veterinary Teaching Hospital; graduate students; veterinary technicians; and new or visiting faculty and researchers. Because CVM faculty, clinicians, and researchers are on twelve-month fiscal year appointments, June, July, and August are typically very busy with library instruction for these groups. Brief orientation sessions for new interns and residents are held upon their arrival in June and July, respectively. These orientations include a brief library tour and a one-page handout outlining basic library services and recommended Web sites and databases. This provides a quick introduction to the HSL until the annual one-hour HSL update session in September. This session, which is designed for all clinicians and house officers, features live database search demonstrations, highlights new features added to the existing core of databases and services, and outlines future plans for upcoming additions to electronic resources and services. At the same time, a range of HSL services, OPAC, and core features of the existing databases are reviewed, in large part for the benefit of those new to WSU. Site addresses for the HSL Web site and relevant library database guides are also provided, in lieu of distributing paper copies that may become outdated quickly or filed away and never used. Graduate students in the Department of Veterinary Microbiology and Pathology take part in a similar session early in the fall semester.

Sessions geared to faculty members and house officers primarily cover new features added to existing core databases such as VETCD/BEASTCD and PubMed, as well as other databases, electronic resources, and tools in the HSL collection. These can include items that have primarily human medicine content, such as full-text medical and pharmacology books, or new resources that make the library's resources easier to use, such as electronic journal collections, SFX context-sensitive reference linking software, or the ILLiad interlibrary loan system.[23]

EVALUATION METHODS

Response to these instructional outreach programs has been overwhelmingly positive. The veterinary librarian is asked to give the sessions every year, and attendance is very good, with many questions asked. Attendees often request an electronic copy of the handout. Catchy titles, including phrases such as "The Library on Your Desktop" and "24/7 Access," help build attendance.

WSU College of Veterinary Medicine students and faculty see the HSL librarians and staff as important partners in the educational process. CVM patrons consistently provide positive responses to the inclusion of information skills in the curriculum and support the acquisition of a growing number of electronic resources. As a result of this close partnership, faculty, staff, and students of the CVM clearly demonstrate their recognition of the importance of the library and its personnel. CVM students and faculty are active participants on the HSL Advisory Committee. Candidates interviewing for veterinary clinical sciences faculty positions at the CVM are scheduled for a half-hour meeting with the veterinary subject specialist, and the library is included in tours for prospective students. HSL librarians are often asked to present a seminar on veterinary information resources at the annual continuing education conference sponsored by the CVM for veterinarians in the region. The CVM recognizes admission to the Academy of Health Information Professionals as equivalent to becoming board certified in a veterinary medical specialty.

CONCLUSION

In summary, successful navigation of electronic databases is seen as a vital component of the veterinary curriculum at Washington State University. Strong liaison relationships demonstrate that students, faculty, and practitioners recognize the importance of both the library and professional librarians. The partnerships between veterinary faculty and librarians allow for experimentation with new instructional techniques. Creative collaboration has had a demonstrated positive effect on student learning.

NOTES

1. Marshall, Joanne Gard, Fitzgerald, Dorothy, and Busby, Lorraine. "A Study of Library Use in Problem-Based and Traditional Medical Curricula." *Bulletin of the Medical Library Association* 81(July 1993):299-305.

2. Sewell, Winifred and Teitelbaum, Sandra. "Observations of End-User Online Searching Behavior Over Eleven Years." *Journal of the American Society for Information Science* 37(July 1986):234-245.

3. Sutcliffe, A.G., Ennis, Mark, and Watkinson, S.J. "Empirical Studies of End-User Information Searching." *Journal of the American Society for Information Science* 51(November 2000):1211-1231.

4. Kaplowitz, Joan R. and Yamamoto, David O. "Web-Based Library Instruction for a Changing Medical School Curriculum." *Library Trends* 50(Summer 2001):47-57.

5. Burrows, Suzetta Cecile and Tylman, Wieslawa T. "Evaluating Medical Student Searches of MEDLINE for Evidence-Based Information: Process and Application of Results." *Bulletin of the Medical Library Association* 87(October 1999): 471-476.

6. Burrows, Suzetta, Moore, Kelly, and Arriaga, Joaquin. "Developing an 'Evidence-Based Medicine and Use of the Biomedical Literature' Component As a Longitudinal Theme of an Outcomes-Based Medical School Curriculum: Year 1." *Journal of the Medical Library Association* 91(January 2003):34-41.

7. Schilling, Katherine, Ginn, David S., and Mickelson, Patricia. "Integration of Information-Seeking Skills and Activities into a Problem-Based Curriculum." *Bulletin of the Medical Library Association* 83(April 1995):176-183.

8. PubMed [electronic resource]. Bethesda, MD: National Library of Medicine, 1966-. Available: <http://www.pubmed.gov/>.

9. AGRICOLA [electronic resource]. Washington, DC: National Agricultural Library, 1970-. Available: <http://agricola.nal.usda.gov/98/>.

10. Pelzer, Nancy L. and Leysen, Joan M. "Use of Information Resources by Veterinary Practitioners." *Bulletin of the Medical Library Association* 79(January 1991):10-16

11. Wales, Tim. "Practice Makes Perfect? Vets' Information Seeking Behaviour and Information Use Explored." *ASLIB Proceedings* 52(July/August 2000): 235-246.

12. Murphy, Sarah Anne. "Applying Methodological Search Filters to CAB Abstracts to Identify Research for Evidence-Based Veterinary Medicine." *Journal of the Medical Library Association* 90(October 2002):406-410.

13. Pelzer, Nancy L. and Leysen, Joan M. "Library Use and Information-Seeking Behavior of Veterinary Medical Students." *Bulletin of the Medical Library Association* 76(October 1988):328-333.

14. Pelzer, Nancy L., Wiese, William H., and Leysen, Joan M. "Library Use and Information-Seeking Behavior of Veterinary Medical Students Revisited in the Electronic Environment." *Bulletin of the Medical Library Association* 86(July 1998):346-355.

15. VETCD [computer file]. Newton Lower Falls, MA: SilverPlatter Information, 1973-. Available: <http://www.ovid.com/>.

16. BEASTCD [computer file]. Newton Lower Falls, MA: SilverPlatter Information, 1973-. Available: <http://www.ovid.com/>.

17. SFX Context Sensitive Linking. Tel Aviv, Israel: ExLibris Corporation, 2001. Available: <http://www.exlibrisgroup.com/resources/sfx/sfx.PDF>.

18. Hines, Stephen A., Eriks, Inge S., and Palmer, Guy H. "An Evolutionary Approach to Curricular Reform: Development of an Integrated Semester and Cross-Disciplinary Simulation." *Journal of Veterinary Medical Education* 22(January 1995):21-25.

19. McCord, Sarah K. DC Literature Search. Pullman, WA: Washington State University, 2001-2003. Available: <http://www.vetmed.wsu.edu/dcgeneral/lit_search.htm>.

20. Washington State University Diagnostic Challenges Planning Committee. DC Home Page. Pullman, WA: Washington State University, 1997-2003. Available: <http://www.vetmed.wsu.edu/dcgeneral/>.

21. Worthley, L.I. "A System-Structured Medical Record for Intensive Care Patient Documentation." *Critical Care Medicine* 3(September-October 1975):188-191.

22. Pelzer, Wiese, and Leysen, "Library Use and Information-Seeking Behavior"; Rankin, Jocelyn A. "Problem-Based Medical Education: Effect on Library Use." *Bulletin of the Medical Library Association* 80(January 1992):36-43.

23. OCLC ILLiad—About. Dayton, OH: OCLC, 2002. Available: <http://www.oclc.org/illiad/about/>.

Chapter 3

Researching the Evidence in Physical Therapy at the University of Missouri–Columbia

Rebecca S. Graves
Evan Prost
Yvette Silvey

SETTING

Established in 1839, the University of Missouri–Columbia enrolls over 24,000 students in 250 undergraduate and 90 graduate programs. It is the main campus in a four-campus state system, and the largest research university in Missouri. The MU Physical Therapy (MU PT) program was established in 1963 and is a part of the School of Health Professions at the University of Missouri–Columbia. After twenty-three years as a unit of the School of Medicine, the School of Health Professions became an autonomous division in December 2000. As Missouri's only state-supported school of health professions on a campus with an academic health center, it is uniquely positioned to educate highly qualified health care professionals committed to fulfilling a mission of improving society through education, service, and discovery in health and rehabilitation sciences.[1] The entry-level master's of physical therapy program offers highly respected researchers and expert clinicians as faculty and uses an innovative curriculum incorporating traditional methods with student-centered problem-based learning.[2]

The mission of MU PT to the state of Missouri is to provide highly qualified students with professional educational experiences that will enable them to contribute to meeting the physical therapy needs of Missourians. The mission to the students includes providing a rich educational foundation that will equip the graduate with the knowledge, principles, skills, and attitudes needed to provide evidence-based care and contribute to the growing body of knowledge that defines the profession.[3] The MU PT academic philosophy states that the maximum development of the individual is sought by offering educational opportunities that develop creative capacities and critical thinking skills; promote independence of inquiry, vision, judgment, and an awareness of the environment of health care; and support clinical competence and confidence.[4] To support the academic missions of the MU Physical Therapy Department, evidence-based practice has been threaded into the curriculum.

The J. Otto Lottes Health Sciences Library supports the School of Medicine, School of Nursing, School of Allied Health, and University Hospital and Clinics. The library has a collection of 242,869 volumes and currently receives 1,194 periodicals pertaining to medicine, nursing, hospital administration, and related fields. The library also has more than 1,125 online periodicals, 100 electronic books, and 146 electronic databases available to patrons through the library Web site. The library currently employs seven professional librarians and thirteen support staff members. In partnership with Information Technology Services (ITS), the library houses a first-floor computer lab with eighteen PCs and a projector for class training. The computer lab is open for student use when not reserved for hands-on workshops. This lab and the additional computers in the commons outside of the lab are maintained by ITS.

BACKGROUND

The MU PT program has paralleled the American Physical Therapy Association's efforts to advance the profession through research and evidence-based clinical decision making.[5] In 1993, the MU PT program first introduced the principles of critiquing and using research in a one credit hour, writing-intensive course. In 1998, this course was extended to three credit hours and titled Evidence Based Practice. The goal was to prepare PT students to be informed consumers of professional research and use the evidence in their clinical decision making.

EDUCATIONAL APPROACHES

Professionals know what good practice should be. Instructors know that students learn over time by doing. Librarians know that research is a hard-won skill best learned as a piece of the overall curriculum. Yet students often fail to incorporate this practice in their work because the lack of compelling reasons to change.

The educational services librarian and physical therapy (PT) faculty provided one-hour library workshops for physical therapy students. These workshops were connected with the current classes but were offered without context to the larger program curriculum. The faculty and librarian alike wanted the students to have lifelong skills, but time was short.

Ten years ago, the PT department began the process of adopting evidence-based practice (EBP) into its curriculum. With this change came a need for a more integrated approach or conscientious instruction in research. This chapter reports curricular changes and how they were used by two PT faculty and the educational services librarian to set the foundations of information literacy.

Starting in 1995, students taking EPB came to the library for a ninety-minute workshop. The workshop covered how to perform basic searches in the following databases using the Ovid interface: CINAHL, MEDLINE, and PsycINFO. The focus of the searching was on PT topics such as orthotics for stroke. Although concepts such as Boolean operators and how to narrow searches were covered, how to limit a search to research articles was not.

Evidence-based practice (EBP) has been defined as "a force for integration, bridging together the often separate domains of research and practice and aiming to further streamline the process of generating new clinical knowledge."[6] The basis of using the evidence in practice evolved from evidence-based medicine.[7] The definitions, principles, and resources of evidence-based medicine have been very helpful, but the focus is different.[8-9] Searching for PT evidence can be cumbersome since the databases focus on medical management. Library services are integral to the foundations of information literacy needed for EBP.

In 2002, the MU Physical Therapy program started to recognize EBP as a philosophy to be woven through the curriculum rather than a concept to be taught once a semester. Based on recommendations gleaned from Boston University's Sargent College of Health and Re-habilitation Sciences, three phases for teaching evidence-based skills and knowledge were introduced and threaded throughout the three-year curriculum.[10] The three phases are described here and presented in Table 3.1.

> *First professional year:* Students will understand the philoso-phy of EBP in their decision-making processes and become familiar with how and where to find the evidence.
>
> *Second professional year:* Students will formally learn how to assess and interpret the evidence in PT 303, *Evidence-Based Practice,* and begin using and communicating the evidence in their clinical decision making.
>
> *Third professional year:* Students will become well-versed in assessing, interpreting, using, and communicating the evi-dence in their clinical decision making to prepare for using best practices. Special emphasis is given to the use of open-access, nonsubscription sources of information retrieval.

In order to equip the students with the knowledge and skills re-quired to find, critique, and communicate the evidence, the need for extended library expertise was recognized. Additional practice of skills and exposure to knowledge were needed to internalize the EBP phi-losophy. Assignments and collaborating workshops were developed for each of the three years of study. The following strategies were de-veloped to carry out the plan's three phases. Library support was an integral part of these efforts.

TABLE 3.1. Teaching evidence-based decision making.

MU PT curriculum	Phase 1	Phase 2	Phase 3
Implemented in program	First professional year	Second professional year	Third professional year
Content	Finding the evidence	Finding the evidence (continued)	Finding the evidence (continued)
		Critiquing and using the evidence	Critiquing and using the evidence (continued)
		Communicating the evidence	Communicating the evidence (continued)

Phase 1

PT 220, Introduction to PT, is the first course in the professional program. Workshop components include Introduction to Evidence-Based Decision Making in PT, Medical Databases, Evidence Based (EB) Tool Kit, and the MU PT Department Web site as the portal to be used to seek and analyze research information for current students and alumni.[11-12]

The focus of the first professional year is to acquaint students with the information resources to be used over the next three years. In the summer semester of their first professional year, a two-hour library workshop introduces them to both EBP and subject databases such as CINAHL, MEDLINE, and PEDro. CINAHL and MEDLINE are searched through the Ovid interface. PEDro is a free database produced by the Centre for Evidence-Based Physiotherapy at the University of Sydney, Australia.

Even though the students may have taken a library skills course in their first two years of undergraduate study, the use of Boolean connectors as well as the difference between searching with text words or subject headings are covered. Truncation or use of wildcards is also touched on when performing a text word search.

Phase 2

The second professional year adds skills of critiquing, using, and communicating the evidence. In the fall semester, the students take PT 303, *Evidence Based Practice,* a writing-intensive course. Writing assignments are designed to further critical thinking and clear communication skills. "Evidence-Based Recommendations" is the final paper and portfolio that culminates the semester-long process of critical thinking, information retrieval and synthesis, and writing. For this course, students attend three sessions at the Health Sciences Library. The first session covers background material such as using electronic texts to find information on disorders and diseases. Three databases (MEDLINE, CINAHL, and PEDro) are reviewed. Additional searching strategies are introduced, such as using publication types and subject headings to limit retrieval to individual research articles. Finally, time is allowed for the students to work on their papers with assistance from the instructor and the librarian.

The second session walks the students through two searches. The examples used are student-generated topics. The librarian performs the searches as if doing them "for real." For example, the librarian uses text word searching to find the subject headings. If no appropriate subject headings are available, various text words are brainstormed and searched. This is in contrast to the more traditional but artificial approach of beginning with an example of known subject headings to show off the features of the database. As in the first session, the students are given time to work on their papers with assistance from the instructor and the librarian.

Although the first two sessions focus on finding research articles, the third session focuses on finding systematic reviews. For a full understanding of the research process, students are shown how to limit searches to retrieve research articles, from which they extrapolate and synthesize the data in order to determine patient care. However, once students are in practice, they probably will not have the time to do the intensive searching necessary to retrieve research articles or to critique their validity and methodology, and will depend on summaries or systematic reviews of the current research. This session delves into the databases and searching techniques needed to limit a search to systematic reviews as well as the differences between traditional narrative reviews and systematic reviews. Databases covered include Cochrane Database of Systematic Reviews, ACP Journal Club, and DARE. As these databases do not have a strong showing in PT, instructors discuss ways to narrow searches to systematic reviews in MEDLINE. PEDro is included as well, as it is solely evidenced based, indexing only systematic reviews, randomized controlled trials, and practice guidelines.

During the second semester of their second professional year, the students take PT 316, *Case Management I*. This course is taught using the problem-based learning (PBL) format through case management of acute and chronic medical and surgical conditions, with emphasis on evidence-based decision making.

PBL is a departure from traditional lecture classes because it emphasizes active, student-centered learning in a small-group format. Students meet for several hours twice a week to work on a case study based to varying degrees on a real patient's history. A faculty member attends the group meeting as a facilitator, offering guidance only when the group needs to focus more closely or broadly. Students develop their own learning needs, clinical questions, and topics that merit deeper exploration of the evidence available. This evidence-based research is conducted between classes and the findings are reported at the next group meeting.

Haynes et al.[13] describe the integration of three domains: research evidence, clinical expertise, and patient preference. Using this model as a conceptual framework, each week's PBL case study is concluded on Friday by a group presentation of the evidence found, analyzed, and evaluated in the light of clinical experience and the applicability to the needs of real-life patients having a diagnosis similar to the patient in the PBL case study. Students employ the population, intervention, comparison group, and outcomes (PICO) format to assist information seeking as well as communicating findings by describing the patients, intervention, and outcomes.[7]

As part of the syllabus, students are supplied with an EB Tool Kit that features Web links to medical databases, authority references, and guideline clearinghouses.[11] This EB Tool Kit also contains strategies for more effective searching, such as the use of Medical Subject Headings (MeSH). The educational services librarian was central to the development of the component of the tool kit that addresses strategies for more effective searching.

Part of the course requires that the students post assignments to WebCT, an electronic course management program. Students receive instruction in using this software in the computer lab at the Health Sciences Library. This session is a collaborative effort by the PT instructor, the librarian, and an instructor from Educational Technology at Missouri (ET@MO). ET@MO is a campus department devoted to assisting faculty in producing Web-based and computer-assisted courses. During the workshop, this instructor demonstrates different methods of uploading and downloading documents to the course Web site, and also the use of the asynchronous chat feature to give feedback to classmates and pose clinically relevant questions.

Although the focus of this session is on the assignments and mastering the WebCT software, it includes a brief review of searching MEDLINE, as one of the assignments is for the students to search for research articles and then post the article citations as well as their critique of the article to the course bulletin board. The librarian also participates in the bulletin board postings and discussions throughout the semester, notes the students' searching strategies and offers instruction and clarification when needed.

Phase 3

To help students continue lifelong learning after graduation, the third year emphasizes the use of only open access, free databases and free electronic journals. This simulates the likely access opportunities that students will have after graduation. The EB Tool Kit supplied with PT 415, *Case Management II,* reflects this goal. As in PT 316, each week culminates in the student presentation of evidence found, analyzed, applied, and communicated to their peers, all within the conceptual framework of the Haynes model.[13]

The students attend their last session at the library during PT 415 in the fall semester of their third professional year. As stated, the students will not be able to access most databases and journals once they have graduated. To enable the students to continue practicing evidence-based PT, they are introduced to PubMed.

By now, it is assumed that students have gained basic searching skills, so the thrust of this session is on how to effectively use PubMed. For many students, it is tempting to trust in the machine by entering text words and accepting the results returned. Instead, the students are shown how to use the Details button to view the search strategy used as well as how to use the MeSH terms to search more accurately. Particularly in PT, students need to be aware of how terms are used. For example, searching "physical therapy AND stroke" will focus more on the specialty of PT as the term maps not to "physical therapy techniques" but to "physical therapy [specialty]." The use of History to combine search sets, Cubby to store search strategies, and Limits to narrow retrieval are also explored.

The final course, PT 416, *Case Management III,* has no corresponding library workshop. However, the students are expected to apply the research skills that they have learned over the previous semesters. This course culminates in a capstone project that is done in lieu of a thesis. Students begin by choosing one of the five case studies they have researched as a group. They create a poster that cites the evidence and references they have found, analyzed, and critiqued. A formal public poster presentation provides the opportunity to communicate evidence-based conclusions to other health professionals and students. The posters are independently judged and submitted for presentation at the annual state convention of the Missouri Physical Therapy Association.

EVALUATION METHODS

In previous years, the workshops were evaluated by an informal survey of the students. They were asked to write down on 3 × 5 cards one thing about the workshop that was beneficial and one thing that could be improved. The majority of comments were positive, for example, stating that the students learned about specific searching techniques such as exploding MeSH terms. However, a few noted that the workshops were too long and that their skills were already adequate.

With the change to the evidence-based curriculum, two evaluations were carried out, one informal and the other formal. Informally, the librarian observed the postings of the students in PT 316 where they had to list their search strategy. Even though it was covered in the workshop for that semester, the students still were missing the correct subject headings in MEDLINE.

The formal evaluation surveyed students in their second year at the end of PT 303. Of the twenty-eight students in the class, seventeen (60 percent) stated that the course had increased their skills of retrieving specific information from scientific databases by 75 to 100 percent. Several commented that the class increased their feelings of comfort and competence. Five stated that they had had no knowledge of available resources or how to use them.

Students were also asked separately if they were competent at critiquing, integrating, and synthesizing relevant literature into their work. They were asked to rate themselves on a scale of one to ten, with ten being very competent. Again the majority, 60 to 78 percent, answered that they were competent to very competent, choosing seven or higher on the Likert scale.

From this survey, the authors were able to identify ongoing challenges with regard to increasing information literacy in EBP. The major challenges include (1) lack of information about literacy competencies; (2) lack of faculty knowledge of new EBP resources; (3) lack of a checks and balances system in place to evaluate library effectiveness in teaching EBP skills; and (4) lack of transfer of knowledge to actual clinical practice.

FUTURE PLANS

The authors have identified a need to develop competencies in the use of databases and search strategies. Although existing workshops represent an improvement over past instruction, content is not sequenced in the most effective manner. For example, to begin by finding research via Ovid databases might be too complex. Students may benefit from first being introduced to the different professional levels of resources such as Web sites, textbooks, and professional journals. Also, students need to be gradually introduced to the complexity of the use of subject headings versus text words. Finally, students need to be introduced to the appropriateness of a five-minute search as opposed to an in-depth literature search.

CONCLUSION

It is the opinion of the authors that the curriculum is rich but lacks systematic checks and balances for faculty and students to periodically verify their accuracy in information literacy. Each curriculum phase needs a formal evaluation of EBP competencies. Ideally, this would be a consistent, standardized evaluation that produces data to compare over time.

The push to use evidence in physical therapy clinical decision making has marked a closer collaboration between the J. Otto Lottes Health Sciences Library and the MU PT Department. This has led to a more integrated information curriculum for the PT students and faculty involved. Although the changes and additions have been positive, ongoing challenges have been identified through the authors' practical experiences.

NOTES

1. University of Missouri–Columbia School of Health Professions: About the School. Columbia, MO: The Curators of the University of Missouri, 2002. Available: <http://www.umshp.org/shpsite/aboutshp.htm>.

2. Physical Therapy at the University of Missouri School of Health Professions: Problem-Based Learning. Columbia, MO: Evan Prost, 2002. Available: <http://www.umshp.org/pt/pbl.htm>.

3. Physical Therapy at the University of Missouri School of Health Professions: About MU PT, Our Mission. Columbia, MO: Evan Prost, 2002. Available: <http://www.umshp.org/pt/mission.htm>.

4. Physical Therapy at the University of Missouri School of Health Professions: About MU PT, Academic Philosophy. Columbia, MO: Evan Prost, 2002. Available: <http://www.umshp.org/pt/educ_philo.htm>.

5. "Challenges 2000." *Magazine of Physical Therapy* 8(January 2000): 43-46.

6. Law, Mary. "Introduction to Evidence-Based Practice." In *Evidence-Based Rehabilitation: A Guide to Practice,* edited by Mary Law. Thorofare, NJ: SLACK Incorporated, 2002, 7.

7. Sackett, D.L., Straus, S.E., Richardson, W.S., Rosenburg, W., and Haynes, R.B. *Evidence-Based Medicine: How to Practice and Teach EBM,* Second Edition. Edinburgh: Churchill Livingstone, 2000.

8. Centre for Evidence-Based Medicine. Headington, UK: Centre for Evidence-Based Medicine, University Department of Psychiatry, Warneford Hospital, 2002. Available: <http://www.cebm.net/>.

9. Centre for Evidence-Based Medicine. Toronto: University Health Network—Mount Sinai Hospital, 2002. Available: <http://www.cebm.utoronto.ca/>.

10. Boston University Center for Rehabilitation Effectiveness. Sargent College of Health and Rehabilitation Sciences. Training Courses Summer Faculty Institute: How to Teach Evidence Based Practice in the Professional Curricula. Boston: Boston University, 2002. Available: <http://www.bu.edu/cre/courses/FacultyInstitute.html>.

11. University of Missouri Tool Kit: Search. Columbia, MO: Evan Prost, 2003. Available: <http://www.missouri.edu/~proste/search.htm>.

12. University of Missouri Tool Kit: Analyze. Columbia, MO: Evan Prost, 2003. Available: <http://www. missouri.edu/~proste/analyze.htm>.

13. Haynes, R. Brian, Sackett, David L., Gray, J. Muir A., Cook, Deborah J., and Guyatt, Gordon. "Transferring Evidence from Research into Practice: 1. The Role of Clinical Care Research Evidence in Clinical Decisions." *ACP Journal Club* 125(November/December 1996):A14-A15.

Chapter 4

The Librarian As Partner in the Development of the Health Care Informatics Curriculum at James Madison University

Jennifer McCabe

SETTING

James Madison University (JMU) is a comprehensive university comprising six colleges with a total 2002-2003 enrollment of 15,612 students. JMU is served by one central library, Carrier Library, and two satellite libraries, the Music Library and the College of Integrated Science and Technology (CISAT) Library. CISAT is geographically separated from the rest of the campus by an interstate highway. Because of this physical separation, the CISAT Library was established to house a library staff, a reference collection, course reserves, and a media center. A delivery service between the CISAT Library and Carrier Library allows for circulation, although no circulating books or journals are housed in the CISAT Library. The virtual and intellectual resources in the CISAT Library have the greatest value to CISAT faculty, students, and staff. These include the electronic databases and program-specific research guides, which are maintained by the two CISAT librarians, and the subject expertise and service orientation of all CISAT Library staff. Two other librarians liaise with CISAT departments but work in the main library.

CISAT departments include Health Science, Nursing, Social Work, Integrated Science and Technology (ISAT), Communication Sciences and Disorders, Kinesiology, Psychology, Computer Science, and Geography. Philosophically, CISAT is unusual in that students are encouraged to engage in research and practica as undergraduates and to glean as much real-world experience as possible prior to graduation. The mission of the college states:

> The College of Integrated Science and Technology encompasses programs of professional education whose common denominator is the use of science and technology to enhance the quality of life in the modern world. The primary mission of the college is to educate students in the areas of the applied sciences, health, technology, and human services.[1]

Because of the departmental composition of the college, interdisciplinary work is encouraged and opportunities cultivated. There is a unique spirit of cooperation in CISAT, where it is commonly accepted that interdisciplinary work prepares students well for future workplace roles.

The mission of the JMU libraries is to connect students and faculty to ideas.[2] Librarians are active participants in the intellectual life of the campus, enjoying faculty status and the opportunity to serve on university committees. The library, like the college, strives to cultivate an atmosphere of innovation and collaboration both interdepartmentally and university-wide.

One of the goals of the General Education program at JMU is to ensure that all students learn effective information-seeking skills. This goal, enforced by the requirement that all freshmen must pass an Information Seeking Skills Test (ISST), is testament to the value placed on information seeking and the degree of integration of the library into the curriculum. In addition to requiring that all students achieve specific competencies in information literacy, many departments participate in an annual assessment of the information-seeking skills of their graduating classes. Notably, the Health Science Department has been assessing their students' skills for years and the Social Work Department has started to do so. This assessment provides a valuable tool for librarians to use as they design and deliver library instruction to various students.

EDUCATIONAL APPROACHES

JMU has a robust and dynamic liaison librarian program. Seventeen librarians act as liaisons to the academic departments on campus. Liaison activities include library instruction, collection development, communicating with departments regarding library matters, writing and updating assessment tests, and various other activities that foster trust and collaboration. The liaison program has been in place since 1986 and serves as the cornerstone of library service to the academic departments.

Library instruction is an essential part of the liaison program, with all librarians participating. During the 2001-2002 academic year, 7,104 students and faculty at JMU received course-related library instruction, in a total of 273 sessions. An additional 3,333 students used *Go for the Gold,* the library's online tutorial.[3] *Go for the Gold* introduces students to library research at JMU and prepares them for the ISST. Librarians also taught semester-long courses, including two sessions on research for honors students and *Introduction to Health Care Informatics for Professionals,* which is described in detail.

Because of the strength of the library instruction program and the institutional commitment to information literacy, the university is recognized as a "Best Practice" institution by the Association of College and Research Libraries. Information literacy programs at "Best Practice" institutions share many of the following ten characteristics, which represent the paragon of such programs:

- A mission statement
- Goals and objectives
- Planning
- Significant administrative and institutional support
- Articulation with the curriculum
- Collaboration among disciplinary faculty, librarians, and other program staff
- Pedagogy
- Staff
- Outreach activities
- Assessment/evaluation of information literacy, including program performance and student outcomes[4]

Identification as a "Best Practice" institution is an indication that the library and its corollary programs enjoy a cooperative and supportive relationship with the university as a whole. Further, librarians are recognized as contributing members of the academic community and valuable resources for curriculum development.

Librarians in the CISAT Library enjoy a unique relationship with the college and individual faculty members. Although not modeled specifically on the college librarian program at Virginia Tech,[5] the relationship is similar. The library and the librarians' offices are located in the same academic building as the departments they serve, allowing library operations to become part of the daily life of the building and the college. Students view librarians as professors, and teaching faculty see librarians as colleagues.

In 2000, a group of CISAT department heads met, with the associate dean of the college as their leader, to identify unmet needs in the undergraduate curriculum. One of the needs was for an introductory informatics class that would allow nursing, health science, social work, and ISAT students to participate. Health informatics is an inherently interdisciplinary subject, as its simplest definition is the application of information technology to enhance patient care. Because each of the identified student cohorts had different information needs and uses, it was thought that each cohort would benefit from a cross-disciplinary approach to the course.

In 2001, a teaching team was identified, composed of one full-time faculty member each from health science, nursing, social work, and ISAT. As goal setting began, the associate dean asked the health and human services librarian, liaison to the health science, nursing, and social work departments, to assist in identifying appropriate reading materials for the class. That librarian began attending curriculum planning meetings, and when the dean felt that the planning had gained enough momentum she stepped out. The dean advised the group to elect a leader to manage the process of developing the course, writing the syllabus, and ensuring that the class met the goals identified by the department heads. The teaching team asked the librarian to join them as faculty in the class and to lend her skills in managing the process.

This was a golden opportunity to align a single class with the information literacy goals of the institution, as well as ensure that information literacy and library instruction were woven seamlessly into the course. Further, because the subject matter dealt with information, opportunities to instruct students on the value of honing their information-seeking and evaluation skills were plentiful. Finally, with a librarian as the leader, the course could be constructed using the best information resources and services that the library offered, often to the surprise and delight of the other teaching faculty.

Managing the development of the informatics course presented a number of challenges. First, participation in the course was intended to mimic the ways that professionals in disparate fields interact with the same information, as well as to identify the information needs unique to each profession. The challenge was to identify an institution that had taken this approach to the subject. This resulted in a need for a great deal of information to be gathered, read, shared, and synthesized into the planning process, a task that the librarian performed with aplomb.

The challenge of student diversity was another strength of the class. It was hoped that student representation would parallel that typically found in a workplace. Initially, the student composition drew almost equally from each major and each grade level. Identifying reading material that was accessible to all and designing assignments that were achievable by all required great effort. Leading the students to common ground proved challenging and rewarding.

Because the course was team taught by five individuals, there was a need to establish a single person as the point of reference. The librarian who had handled the administrative creation of the course, stepped up as the first person for students to contact with questions and concerns. She also coordinated communication between the other teaching faculty and called meetings when major decisions needed to be made. After the semester began, the faculty met face to face only once more, to arrive at a consensus on the final grades at the end of the semester.

Initially the syllabus (see Appendix A) was mapped out with appropriate faculty assuming responsibility for lectures in their areas of expertise. When they had specific articles or book chapters, those were included. When they did not, the librarian was able to search for appropriate material. In setting up the syllabus, two class periods were devoted to the concept of information literacy and its relationship to health literacy and the larger informatics picture. Additional lab time was scheduled for targeted library instruction, from both a practitioner's point of view and a student's point of view. Patient education material was compared to research material, and the utility of both was discussed. The librarian offered all of the information literacy content and library instruction.

After a historical introduction to the study of informatics, the librarian designed the information literacy exercise (Box 4.1). It demonstrates to the students how information literacy is related to health literacy and how essential it is to both patients and caregivers. Students read and discussed case studies in which patients in various situations have a range of information needs. The case studies were chosen to highlight language barriers, age barriers, point of view barriers, and a diversity of available technology. After the patients' needs were discussed, other information needs were examined. Each time, the students were asked to comment on the sources of information, determine who needs it, and how they will know it is authoritative. The

---

BOX 4.1. Information Literacy Exercise

Goal of the Exercise

The students will understand that information literacy is the ability to identify an information need, find the relevant information, evaluate the information for authority, and apply it to a situation. They will demonstrate the ability to identify information needs and isolate potential sources of information pertaining to particular cases.

Students will work in small groups. Read the case study and identify the people involved in the scenario. Discuss the kinds of information each person needs and where he or she might get it. Be creative; think about what happened before and after the case. Choose one person from the case and answer the following questions from his or her perspective. After answering these questions each case will be discussed with the class.

What is your role? _____

1. What is the most important information you need to get?
2. Where can you get this information?
3. How will you know that the information is authoritative?
4. What will you do with the information once you have it?
5. Did your colleagues raise any new issues that you might not have thought of?

goal of the session was to illustrate the variety of kinds of information different people need about the same topic.

To discuss information literacy in the context of patient education and bibliographic research, students were asked to read "The Patient Informatics Consult Service (PICS): An Approach for a Patient Centered Service,"[6] which describes an early information prescription program at Vanderbilt University. The librarian led the discussion, in which students were asked to identify issues related to the prescription of information for various health conditions. The goal of this session was to continue to think about the different ways information can be organized and delivered, and how the same information can be presented in various ways. After the discussion, students were given a prescription (see Box 4.2) and guided through the use of various library databases to fill it. Since all students in the class had basic orientation to the library, either online or through practice, most of this lab time was spent using health databases.

In addition to delivering a number of lectures and leading discussions, the librarian brings added expertise to this particular class due to the subject matter. The study of informatics includes examining human computer interaction, database design and maintenance, and the role of controlled vocabularies in the context of health care and medicine. Librarians have been studying these issues and integrating them into their work for many years. The first controlled vocabulary that most students use is probably subject headings, and it is usually introduced to them by librarians. Likewise, most students have experience searching the library databases, as well as a rudimentary understanding of their architecture. Using examples that students know helps them to understand other applications of the technology. Finally, most public service librarians today strive to help users understand how to use computer applications as tools for their research. In doing so, they gain a practical understanding of the various ways in which people interact with machines.

Blackboard was used to manage the course content. Blackboard is a Web-based course management system whereby instructors can set up Web pages for individual classes and make resources available to the enrolled students. Because there were five instructors, organization of their content was a paramount concern. The librarian used

Blackboard to post the syllabus and create individual folders for each instructor. These folders eventually contained readings or links to library resources, lecture notes, and other external links. The use of Blackboard became an essential element of the class. In addition to managing content, it allowed for online communication, both synchronous and asynchronous as well as electronic submission of assignments.

BOX 4.2. Library Research Lab Exercise

Read "Patient Informatics Consult Service (PICS): An Approach for a Patient Centered Service" by Williams, MD et al. in Bull Med Libr Assoc 89(April 2001):185-193.

Examine the prescription you have been given and identify the main information needs. Using the following databases, identify one article (or Web site where appropriate) that addresses the information needs. Please hand in the assignment when you are finished.

Health and Wellness Resource Center
CINAHL
PubMed
MEDLINEplus

Sample Information Prescriptions:

- Sixty-two-year-old postmenopausal woman recently diagnosed with type 2 diabetes. Needs information about dietary and lifestyle changes. English not first language; prefers material in Spanish if possible.
- Eighteen-year-old female athlete, diagnosed with acute lateral epicondylitis. Needs exercises and management information.
- Thirty-seven-year-old male, hypertensive, obese. Needs information on smoking cessation, stress management, and dietary changes.
- Marginally illiterate parents of twenty-three-month-old child. Child is newly diagnosed with epilepsy. Parents need information on drug compliance, record keeping, and seizure care.
- Twenty-two-year-old Somali immigrant, male with chronic depression. Recently switched to 150 mg Effexor for management. Needs easy-to-read information on side effects of drug, and record keeping.

EVALUATION METHODS

Blackboard courseware was also used as an evaluation tool. Because of experience with the concept of assessment, and because of the need to get very specific information from the students, the librarian set up the evaluations, which were delivered in the form of anonymous online surveys. Rather than the traditional Likert scale used widely in higher education, students were asked to describe the course content in their own words and to rate the class activities according to learning accomplished. Based on survey results, the class was modified slightly the second semester. Most notably, instead of using the textbook the second time the class was offered, journal articles were assigned instead.

The class has been offered successfully three times to interdisciplinary groups of students. The librarians' involvement has had myriad benefits. Most significantly, the traditional relationship between the librarian and the academic departments is stronger. It also resulted in the librarian being invited to serve on an additional college-wide steering committee to plan a new informatics center.

Spending an entire semester with the same group of students proved to be invaluable, offering insight into the lives of undergraduate students, and revealing ways to reach them with library resources. Perhaps most important, the librarian was able to lead by example, exposing the teaching faculty to library services and the students to resources for their work.

The building in which the course is taught (and the library is located) has an operational wireless network. Students routinely connect their laptop computers to the network to do their work and access the library Web and research databases. Involvement in the class presented an interesting incidental opportunity for the library to investigate the application of some new technology. During the third semester the course was offered, a pilot program was instituted that issues personal digital assistants (PDAs) for use with specific class assignments.

The handheld devices are owned by the library, which monitors their use with an eye toward the future. Because PDAs are widely used in health care, and because the informatics class focuses on information technology and the differing information needs and challenges faced in the health care workplace, the choice to pilot the program with the informatics class was an easy one. The issue for the teachers and students is whether students can learn to use this emerging technology for information retrieval and management in a meaningful way. To this end, an assignment was designed to measure the student use of the device and recognition of its place in the information infrastructure (see Box 4.3). The issue for the library is whether they can manage a collection of devices, which technical, procedural, and intellectual issues arise, and how services may be expanded by using this technology.

BOX 4.3. Informatics for Health Care Professionals Team Project

All health care facilities and people working in them have information needs. These needs vary from person to person and between types of facility. It is incumbent on everyone working in health care to be able to access the information they need and record the information they gather accurately and efficiently.

Your assignment is to use the information presented in class, as well as research done outside of class, to plan the integration of handheld devices into the chosen organization. Each team will present their plan to the class at the end of the semester, as well as submitting a written document describing the plan. Specifically, you must:

1. Select *one* of the following health sector frameworks:
   a. a 250-bed community hospital
   b. a stand-alone not-for-profit skilled nursing facility (120 beds)
   c. an independent (stand-alone) proprietary home health agency
   d. a twelve-physician multispecialty group practice
2. Outline the major and minor issues that you will try to address/resolve by implementing the new technology.
3. Structure how the key health informatics needs of the different health care sectors (clinical, administrative, social work, and information technology) can be rectified.
4. Develop a plan to integrate handheld computers for a *specific use* among the individual cohorts (i.e., clinical staff, social workers, and management) in the facility. Each of the facilities has multiple unfulfilled information needs. Choose the one you feel would be best served by the new hardware and software, and explain why you chose it.

(continued)

(continued)

To guide you along, consider the following for managing the project:

- Create a timeline for tasks and deliverables.
- Manage people/staff (including the composition of the team).
- Manage the budget.
- Identify potential problems that could be encountered at any stage and suggest possible solutions.
- Discuss necessary communication skills and lines of communication.
- Describe the coordination of skills across the team to complete the integration.
- Explain how the project will be monitored and evaluated.
- Choose a device to purchase (model and operating system) and accompanying software application(s) based on what is available right now.
- Discuss how staff will be trained, including how long it will take, who will do it, the user's diversity of attitudes and abilities, and technical support.

CONCLUSION

Involving the librarian in the development of the informatics course has been mutually beneficial to the college and the library. It is a natural extension of the core values of the profession of librarianship, and possibly offers a glimpse into the future. The paradox in academic librarianship is that as resources increase, physical interaction decreases. Gate counts shrink as resources grow. Given this situation, it is logical that college and university librarians are spending more time in the classroom.

The kind of collaboration described in this chapter represents a paradigm shift in the practice of academic librarianship. Librarians are moving from the role of helper to the role of contributor, a change that should be welcomed by library and campus administration, as it makes available a new pool of talent for the ultimate goal of preparing students for their futures.

APPENDIX: INFORMATICS FOR HEALTH CARE PROFESSIONALS SYLLABUS

Course Description

This course is a multidisciplinary introduction to informatics in health care focusing on technology, data information, and knowledge, and their applications in health care. Emerging trends and issues are examined.

Goals of the Course

At the conclusion of the course the student will be able to do the following:

1. Understand roles of the patient and the health care team as related to health informatics
2. Participate in collaborative cross-role activities with other health and human service disciplines
3. Describe elements of the health care system (settings, types of care, reimbursement mechanisms, finances, delivery of care)
4. Examine issues and challenges facing the health care system (patient rights, confidentiality, quality, access, cost, security)
5. Describe categories of terminology relevant to informatics in the health care system
6. Define and delineate types of information and health information systems
7. Understand the unique challenges of applying information technology to health information
8. Describe legal, ethical, policy, and procedural issues (including privacy and security) related to the design and use of health care information systems
9. Understand how health information systems are designed, implemented, evaluated, and procured
10. Understand how health data are designed, stored, accessed, used, communicated, and archived by various members of the health care team
11. Access and assess health care information and resources on the Internet
12. Examine the anatomy, physiology, and pathophysiology of information technology

---

This document contains the basic elements of the syllabus as distributed to the students. Information specific to JMU, CISAT, and individual faculty members has been deleted. Dates have also been removed.

13. Describe emerging trends in technology within the health care system
14. Understand how data and data systems are used to support analysis and decision making

Course Schedule

Week 1: Introduction to the faculty and history of health care informatics

Week 2: Personal digital assistants (PDAs) and the nursing piece of informatics

Week 3: The social work piece of informatics and the health administration piece

Week 4: Databases; their design and utility

Week 5: Information literacy in health care and bibliographic database searching

Week 6: PDA use in the health care workplace and administrative and clinical decision making

Week 7: Information ethics and technical standards and coding

Week 8: Accreditation and HIPAA

Week 9: Human-computer interaction and research

Week 10: E-health trends and the electronic health record

Week 11: Data gathering and analysis

Week 12: Choosing and implementing a health information system

Week 13: Reserved for final project

NOTES

1. College of Integrated Science and Technology Mission Statement. Harrisonburg, VA: James Madison University, 2003. Available: <http://www.jmu.edu/cisat/mission.htm>.

2. James Madison University Mission Statement. Harrisonburg, VA: James Madison University, 2002. Available: <http://www.lib.jmu.edu/plan/mission.html>.

3. Cameron, Lynn. *Library Instruction Annual Report.* Harrisonburg, VA: James Madison University, 2002.

4. Characteristics of Programs of Information Literacy That Illustrate Best Practices. Chicago, IL: American Library Association, 2003. Available: <http://www.ala.org/ala/acr/acr/standards/characteristics.htm>.

5. Schillie, Jane E., Young, Virginia E., and Ariew, Susan A. "Outreach Through the College Librarian Program at Virginia Tech." *Reference Librarian* 71(2000):71-78.

6. Williams, M. Dawn, Gish, Kimbra Wilder, Guise, Nunzia B., and Carrel, Donna L. "The Patient Informatics Consult Service (PICS): An Approach for a Patient Centered Service." *Bulletin of the Medical Library Association* 89(April 2001):185-193.

Chapter 5

Educating Users of the Health Sciences Library System at the University of Pittsburgh

Linda M. Hartman

SETTING

The University of Pittsburgh's Health Sciences Library System (HSLS) supports education, research, and patient care activities of the University of Pittsburgh's Schools of the Health Sciences and the University of Pittsburgh Medical Center (UPMC) Health System. Three libraries serve this population: Falk Library, WPIC Library, and UPMC Shadyside Library.

Falk Library is located in the hospital complex that serves the academic medical center and the six schools of the health sciences: dentistry, pharmacy, medicine, nursing, public health, and health and rehabilitation sciences. The UPMC Health System consists of more than twenty hospitals, the farthest being 110 miles from Pittsburgh. Some hospitals within the UPMC Health System have librarians on site. The hospitals without a librarian on the premises receive library services and end user training from the coordinator of affiliated hospital services of the HSLS. The coordinator also acts as a liaison between the library system and those librarians at the various hospitals. Each affiliated institution contracts for particular databases and services.

WPIC Library is situated in the Western Psychiatric Institute and Clinic (WPIC) across the street from Falk Library. WPIC is part of the Department of Psychiatry of the University of Pittsburgh School of Medicine. Its members conduct education, research, and critical care. The library's patron base consists of undergraduates, medical students, interns, researchers, postdoctoral students, and clinicians.

Two miles from the Falk and WPIC libraries, UPMC Shadyside Hospital's library consists of two libraries housed together. One library serves the physicians, residents, nurses, and staff, and the other is open to hospital patients and members of the health system in general.

Falk Library employs more than fifteen instructors, including the Computer Media Center (CMC) staff. The CMC staff conducts classes on basic software, such as Photoshop and PowerPoint, and provide support and instruction for personal digital assistants (PDAs). WPIC Library has three instructors who participate in scheduled classes. WPIC librarians are part of the core group who teach MEDLINE, but they also teach classes on finding mental health resources and testing instruments. Specific classes for psychiatry residents have been designed to give in-depth database instruction as needed for their studies. UPMC Shadyside has two instructors who teach MEDLINE, consumer health information, and an overview of library resources. A librarian liaison is assigned to each of the schools of dentistry, pharmacy, nursing, public health, and health and rehabilitation sciences. The WPIC librarians serve as the liaisons for psychiatry personnel.

EDUCATIONAL APPROACHES

Because HSLS serves such a large and diverse patron base, instruction must be diverse and far-reaching. Learning styles, work times, and physical location are factors in the ability of patrons to participate. Some people can learn to use a database on their own, without formal instruction. HSLS provides basic MEDLINE search information in pamphlet form on the literature racks in each library. Database tutorials are accessible through the HSLS Web site <http://www.hsls.pitt.edu/services/instruction/online>.

For patrons who prefer more formal instruction, HSLS offers classes on various days and times. The introduction class involves a detailed tour of the library and instruction on PITTCat, the library's online catalog, and a quick review of the Web site and available databases. This class and other formal classes are published in the Schedule of Classes <http://www.hsls.pitt.edu/services/instruction/calendar>. Other scheduled classes cover searching MEDLINE; using bibliographic management software; finding resources on the World Wide Web; and researching specific topics such as molecular biology and genetics, basic sciences, complementary and alternative medicine, medical humanities, and evidence-based literature. These classes are in addition to the software training offered by the CMC and the mental health-related courses offered by WPIC librarians.

The schedule of classes covers four months at a time. Some classes are offered only once a semester while others are offered multiple times. Printed copies of the schedule are available in each of the libraries, and in the newsletters for the library and hospital system. Fliers describing newer courses are available near the reference desk. Box 5.1 features an example of a library handout.

Classes are held mostly during the week, Monday through Friday. Attendance did not justify continuing to schedule classes on Saturdays. At one time preregistration was required, but this practice was discontinued because people would sign up and then not attend.

The training sessions discussed so far have been held for relatively small groups of people, ranging from one or two per class up to fifteen per session. Larger groups (100 people or more) are accommodated through open houses that last approximately two hours. In late summer, separate open houses are held for the schools of medicine, pharmacy, dentistry, and public health. Each class is divided into groups that rotate between the various library departments: circulation, history of medicine, reference, and CMC. The attendees' final stop is at the refreshments table.

Nursing students receive orientation over several sessions held at the nursing school rather than during an open house. The open house for the new physical therapy students is in early summer. The other departments in the school of health and rehabilitation sciences schedule less formal orientations. These are primarily a tour of the library and CMC as well as a session on basic MEDLINE searching. If a database is specific to the discipline, such as OT Search, it is also included in this first session.

The circulation department oversees the course reserves, on-site storage of older journals, and the photocopiers. The photocopiers accept cash as well as VendaCards. Although there is a minimal charge for these cards, they do reduce the per-page cost of photocopying. They are also required for printing from the library's computers. Circulation is also the point of contact during the evening and on Sunday

---

BOX 5.1. Sample Handout

Health Sciences
Library System
New Class

Basic Science
Information
Resources

This class is designed for basic science researchers who need specialized information in topics such as microbiology, biochemistry, biotechnology, and genetics. The **Biological Abstracts, Chemical Abstracts (SciFinder Scholar)** and **ISI Web of Science** databases will be highlighted as well as tips on how best to use **MEDLINE** to find basic science information. This class is approved for AMA Category 2 CME credit. This is a walk-in class—no registration is required. Attendance is limited to UPMC and University of Pittsburgh faculty, staff, and students.

Class Dates and Times:

	Monday, June 16	10:00-11:30 am
	Thursday, July 24	1:00-2:30 pm

Location:

Falk Library, (200 Scaife Hall), CMC Classroom 2

For more information on these and other classes contact the reference department:
Phone: **412-648-8796**
E-mail: **medlibq@pitt.edu**
or visit our Web site:
http://www.hsls.pitt.edu
and click on "Instruction"

Searching MEDLINE on Ovid
Searching MEDLINE on PubMed

Wednesday, June 4	1:00-2:30 pm
Tuesday, May 20	1:00-2:30 pm
Monday, July 7	2:00-3:30 pm
Tuesday, June 3	9:00-10:30 am

Advanced MEDLINE Searching on Ovid

Thursday, May 29	1:00-2:30 pm

---

when the reference department is closed. Each open house participant receives a free VendaCard. Since the circulation department is responsible for the cards, they distribute them during the open house.

HSLS has a history of medicine collection with 17,000 volumes dating from 1496 to the present. The collection is overseen by the history of medicine librarian, who greets the students and explains the services available to them during affiliation with the university. The students are encouraged to include historical perspectives in research papers written for various courses.

The CMC staff shows the many tools and types of hardware, such as scanners, available for use by HSLS patrons. They also make the students aware of the policies, procedures, and rules and regulations associated with the privileges and responsibilities of using the CMC's resources. HSLS requires logins and passwords to enter the network. During their stop in the CMC, the new students complete applications for their user accounts.

Reference librarians welcome the new students and give a quick introduction to the online catalog as well as other resources available. More in-depth searching instruction is given later. Experience has shown that including search specifics during orientation can result in information overload. Students retain searching instruction more readily when it relates to specific class assignments or research needs.

Because much information is communicated in a short time during these orientation sessions, the participants are given information packets including several items. A fact sheet lists library hours, policies on photocopying and document delivery, pertinent phone numbers, and a brief explanation of resources and services available. A map shows the location of the books in reference, history of medicine, oversize shelves, nursing collection, and general collection.

Many people prefer to do their research from home. Although the university provides faculty, staff, and students with a computer account and dial-up access, this service can get busy at times, making access difficult or very slow. For this reason, many people use an outside Internet service provider. HSLS also provides remote access for users outside the university network. An HSLS Online Account is needed for this and can be obtained by completing the application included in the packet, which includes instructions for accessing HSLS resources through the university account or remotely. Remote access is also useful when clinical tours take patrons outside the university or UPMC system, as they can still access the needed resources.

Other subjects covered by the information packet include searching PITTCat, accessing electronic books and journals, and using the various databases. Most resources have a fact sheet that outlines the subjects covered, publications included, and access instructions.

Everything discussed to this point is arranged by the library or through departmental representatives contacting the library in advance. Times are agreed upon and in the case of the open houses, the number of attendees expected. Questions do arise, however, as one conducts research or attempts to complete assignments. In these instances, patrons either call or come to the reference desk for assistance.

Although most questions at the reference desk can be answered quickly, some can become rather involved. When this occurs, the librarian suggests that the patron return at an appointed time to further discuss the information desired. This practice led to the creation of the consultation service. Parties interested in very specific questions or an in-depth discussion on a topic contact the consultation service coordinator, who assigns librarians to each case on a rotating basis. The librarian then contacts the interested party to gather details of the question and to schedule a time to meet. Consultations can lead to class instruction. After sitting with a liaison for a couple of hours, one faculty member realized there were many aspects of searching particular databases of which she and her co-researchers were not aware. This led to an advanced searching session for faculty of the school.

Professors in the different schools contact their liaison to provide instruction to their students. Generally this involves MEDLINE, PITTCat, and e-journal access. Variations include hands-on instruction in the library's computer lab, hands-on instruction in the school's computer lab, or PowerPoint presentations given in a lecture room. A brief tour of the library is generally included if the students come to the library for searching instruction.

When time permits, the liaisons give the students exercises based on the tours and instruction. The exercises might include searching for particular items on PITTCat or MEDLINE or physically finding items in the library. The scavenger hunt requires the student to find a certain page in a book or journal and write down the answer to a particular question.

All of the instruction thus far described has involved face-to-face contact with the patron. Brief user education takes place over the phone at the reference desk or by the liaison when a patron has a problem or question. However, it is not always possible for the patron to pick up the phone to ask the question. The library may be closed or it may be easier to write out the problem and ask the question. To handle these situations, Ask-a-librarian links are available from the library's Ovid databases. Most of these concern searches on a particular database. For general questions, patrons use a link from the reference Web page. A useful aspect of Ovid's Ask-a-librarian link is the ability to include the search strategy and database being searched. This allows the librarian responding to see the terms being searched, as well as any other pertinent clues.

EVALUATION METHODS

Periodically, attendance figures are reviewed for the scheduled classes. Those classes with few or no attendees are removed from the schedule. For some classes, a brief course description is included along with the instructor's contact information. Those who are interested in the class can make arrangements with the instructor for a one-on-one session or a more formal class for larger groups.

HSLS continuously reviews the courses offered. New databases are added to the collection and veteran databases may change focus or search features. As certain topics, such as molecular biology and genetics, are emphasized in the curricula, the need to find information in these subject areas increases. A molecular biology and genetics information specialist recently joined HSLS. As a result, classes such as Sequence Similarity Searching and *Information Hubs for Molecular Biology and Genetics* have been added to the schedule of classes.

Information seekers are becoming more sophisticated. Courses such as *Introduction to Netscape* once had several participants per session. Today most HSLS users understand how to navigate the more widely used browsers. As a result, this class is no longer offered.

Advanced MEDLINE was added to the schedule because although many users had been searching MEDLINE for some time, they did not always use the database to its fullest potential. *Advanced MEDLINE* takes the searcher beyond the basic subject search and delves into keyword searching, truncation, and exploring the MeSH tree to see if broader and narrower terms can be used.

Some instructors welcome feedback on the sessions they conduct. One librarian compiled an evaluation form and placed it a shared drive accessible to librarians. The two-page evaluation form (see Box 5.2) is meant to be a template with specific questions and open-ended questions. Instructors can choose the preferred format.

Box 5.2. Evaluation Form Template

CONTENT

Goals and objectives were made clear.
Agree/Somewhat Agree/Somewhat Disagree/Disagree

Achieved the objectives as stated.
Agree/Somewhat Agree/Somewhat Disagree/Disagree

I now know how to get started using the information resources demonstrated in this class.
Fully Understand/Somewhat Understand/Still Don't Know

Today's session will help me with my course work.
Agree/Somewhat Agree/Somewhat Disagree/Disagree

FORMAT

Class content was organized and sequenced to make topic understandable.
Agree/Somewhat Agree/Somewhat Disagree/Disagree

Explanations and examples were clear.
Agree/Somewhat Agree/Somewhat Disagree/Disagree

Length of class.
Too Long/Just Right/Too Short

Pace of class.
Too Fast/Just Right/Too Slow

PRESENTER

Presenter demonstrated an understanding of topic.
Agree/Somewhat Agree/Somewhat Disagree/Disagree

Handled audience questions.
Satisfactorily/Unsatisfactorily

Presenter showed how the concepts have practical application.
Agree/Somewhat Agree/Somewhat Disagree/Disagree

OVERALL

Overall score.
Excellent/Good/Fair/Poor

Overall, I am satisfied with what I learned.
Agree/Somewhat Agree/Somewhat Disagree/Disagree

(continued)

(continued)

OPEN-ENDED QUESTIONS

- How would you improve this session?
- Please list 3 important points you learned:
  1.
  2.
  3.
- What did you hope or need to learn from this session?
- Did the session meet these goals and/or needs?
- If not, why not?
- What was most helpful about this training?
- What was the least helpful?

Usually there is consensus among the survey respondents. Sometimes, however, half the group will say the pace was too fast and the other half will say it was just right. The same split decision can occur with the length of the class; some feel it is too long and others say it is just right. On at least one occasion, review of the responses to this question prompted contact with the professor. The librarian suggested splitting the three-hour session, covering many different databases and topics, into two sessions. It would help to alleviate the students' feeling of becoming overwhelmed by the mountain of information being presented to them.

Although no formal analysis has been done of the evaluation responses, the information provided gives the instructor an idea of how the material was received by the students. This can be particularly helpful when a new class has been developed or a new group of students is participating. Undergraduates, graduate students, clinicians, and researchers bring varying amounts of experience to class, which can make a difference in understanding the material presented.

CONCLUSION

New databases and software products appear every day. Some require a very specific knowledge base, such as those dealing with molecular biology or genetics. The databases designed for the clinician or health care consumer may have simple search interfaces, more like those of search engines. On the surface, these do not require as much subject-specific knowledge as those with a more complicated interface. The idea is that the user can simply type in a search statement using terms that may or may not be subject headings. It is not always apparent, however, what terms are being searched. A term could be searched as a subject heading and keyword, giving a much larger set of citations and overwhelming the user. Some interfaces automatically explode subject headings, again giving large numbers of hits. This can also leave the user wondering why certain terms are included in the search results.

Usually, the subject headings further down the MeSH tree are included in the mystery citations. If the user does not have a complete understanding of how the search has been done and/or of the tree structures, the results can be more confusing than helpful. On the other hand, some users simply want results—the answers to a quick and dirty search. It goes back to the idea of precision and recall.

The librarians' job as instructors is to create a balance between these approaches. Going into detail when the user is not interested or does not need it is as dangerous as not giving the detail when it is needed. After the first few minutes, users will tune out the instructor and plod along on their own. This is worse than if they had not come for instruction at all, because now they may be reluctant to come to the library and ask for assistance the next time.

Clinicians, researchers, undergraduates, and graduate students all have specific information needs and unique circumstances requiring the gathering of information. This diverse patron base creates challenges yet offers opportunities to provide end user education. As a result, the HSLS develops a wide variety of training sessions given in several formats and locations.

Chapter 6

Hardin Library for the Health Sciences: Experiencing Change

Denise H. Britigan
Anne K. Gehringer

INTRODUCTION

Hardin Library for the Health Sciences at the University of Iowa has seen dramatic changes in the ways patrons access resources as well as the types of information now available. What was once a repository for print information has become a gateway to countless databases, online journals, and electronic resources. The days of mediated searching have largely come and gone. Patrons themselves are now the primary searchers of online databases such as MEDLINE and CINAHL. This change has challenged librarians to emphasize information literacy skills. At Hardin Library, the increased importance of user education has prompted changes in services, staff, and technology. It has become clear that Hardin Library will need to constantly evolve to stay in touch with the academic and medical needs of its patron base. What follows is a brief account of dealing with the changing roles of librarians to best meet the needs of its clientele.

SETTING

Hardin Library for the Health Sciences serves the research, educational, and clinical needs of the health sciences campus of the University of Iowa. The university is home to almost 30,000 students as well as 11,958 faculty and staff.[1] Situated adjacent to the University of Iowa Hospitals and Clinics as well as a Veterans Administration (VA)

Medical Center, the four-story library building houses 362,185 monographs (including government publications), 2,358 current print journal subscriptions, 2,306 electronic journal subscriptions, and 122 publicly accessible computer workstations.[2]

As part of the University of Iowa Libraries system, which includes thirteen libraries, Hardin Library employs nine professional librarians, two computer support specialists, twelve library assistants and support personnel, and approximately sixteen full-time equivalent (FTE) student workers. Among the many services offered at the library, there is a renewed interest and emphasis in the area of education. Library administration has committed resources and energy to expend and improve the education program at Hardin, including orientations, skills workshops, and course-integrated instruction.

BACKGROUND

In the late 1960s and early 1970s, online databases such as the National Library of Medicine's MEDLINE were introduced. Initially, it was a complex and command-driven process to search these databases for bibliographic records. Librarians often engaged in intensive training sessions to learn the intricacies of a given system. Like many similar institutions, Hardin Library began to offer its patrons access to these databases through mediated searching. A special room was set aside for this process and patrons reserved times to sit one-on-one with a librarian who was skilled in online searching. Patrons offered input into the types of information they desired while the librarians manipulated the computer. For those accustomed to using *Index Medicus,* this new electronic environment was exciting as well as a time-saver.

For many years, Hardin librarians continued to offer mediated searching on a fee basis. By the 1980s, the number of databases available had grown exponentially, requiring librarians to become knowledgeable about many different search interfaces. The mid-1980s saw a change that revolutionized the way patrons gained access to electronic databases. The first CD-ROM version of MEDLINE was produced, which enabled Hardin Library to set aside one public terminal dedicated to searching those preloaded resources. Patrons could reserve a time to use the computer and perform their MEDLINE searches directly. Although mediated searching remained an option, many patrons relished the ability to direct their own research. What quickly became obvious to librarians, however, was that enthusiasm and a medical background alone did not a searcher make. Several studies have found that enduser searching produces less effective results than searches performed by librarians.[3-4]

EDUCATIONAL APPROACHES

Hardin Library soon responded to the increasing reliance on personal computers by creating a cluster of workstations for the public to use. Around the same time, the World Wide Web emerged and created a stir of activity among academicians and students alike. The small computer lab in Hardin soon became a place of interest to many people seeking to explore the vast resources of the Internet. One of the librarians had been assigned to oversee the computers and had an office located adjacent to the workstations. He began to offer lunchtime training sessions for patrons interested in improving their Internet searching skills. Word spread and soon he provided tutorials to groups of people crowded around a single terminal. Although Hardin librarians had always provided the traditional tours and orientations to their building, this was the first time that instruction in an electronic environment had taken place.

Around that time, several other librarians began to give instructional sessions to groups of students likely to use MEDLINE or CINAHL for their research. This was before the age of Internet-wired classrooms. Instructors used overhead transparencies to show screen shots of the various databases being demonstrated. It was a labor-intensive process for librarians to prepare these lessons as well as for the students to sit in the audience and absorb the information passively. Students receiving hands-on instruction in using electronic resources retain more information than those exposed to only a lecture or demonstration of the same resources.[5]

For several years, the staff of Hardin Library continued to offer formal instruction to groups of patrons as well as more informal tutoring to patrons using the library's computers. Gradually, the number of online databases grew and their search interfaces became easier to navigate. It was clear that patrons desired access to these resources and increasingly wanted to be the ones directly responsible for finding bibliographic information.

Up until this point, Hardin Library did not have a librarian whose primary responsibility was user education. All of the reference librarians had shared in the instruction process, some providing more time and interest than others. Eventually, an experienced librarian was brought on board to oversee the education program. This individual worked with the health sciences faculty to promote library education and to continue the traditional bibliographic instruction that was being offered.

In March 1995, a strategic planning effort resulted in a report titled *Meeting Information Needs of the Health Professions at the University of Iowa*. The jointly appointed Hardin Library Strategic Planning Group was composed of faculty and staff from the health sciences, along with librarians, and was chaired by the head of the Hardin Library. Based on this report, the staff members of Hardin Library developed an implementation plan. The plan was used to guide efforts on "expanding user education, installing an Information Arcade [public computer lab] in Hardin Library, strengthening on-line information resources, increasing outreach and grant-funded activities, and providing health sciences information via the Hardin Library home page on the World Wide Web site."[6]

Hardin Library responded to this challenge by creating the Information Commons, a state-of-the-art computing facility. The Information Commons East was completed in 1996 and West in 1999. This facility now houses forty-seven public terminals, several high-end multimedia workstations, and two fifty-seat computer classrooms. While the patrons marveled at the available computers, the electronic classrooms excited the librarians. Gone were the days of overhead transparencies or a single Internet-connected computer. Students could now receive their group instruction at the library. Each student could sit at his or her own workstation and practice the skills that were being taught. Overhead projection screens allowed all in the room to view exactly what the instructor was doing on his or her computer. Group instruction was truly transformed. Students could now engage in an active process that enabled them to gain hands-on experience with a given resource. Soon practically all educational offerings were given in the Information Commons.

Interestingly, while Hardin Library saw changes in its facility, it also witnessed frequent librarian turnover in user education. The original librarian hired for this job left after two years and was followed by a few other professionals. During several extended periods, in fact, the position remained vacant. Finally, in 2002, a number of organizational changes took place in the library. A new director was hired, as was a new assistant director for public services. Several temporary librarians had provided most of the instruction until one was finally hired on a permanent basis in the latter half of 2002. She was soon followed by the addition of another new librarian. It was decided that one of these new librarians would be in charge of reference while the other would oversee education. Once again, Hardin Library had a permanent staff member who could focus on modifying and improving the library's educational offerings.

The education program at Hardin Library includes instructional handouts, open-enrollment workshops, tailored workshops, walk-in consultations, scheduled consultations, and course-integrated instruction. Each of these offerings contributes to the wide array of services available to meet the information needs of the patrons. These areas will be examined in terms of their current status, need for improvement, methods used to improve them, and findings based on these methods.

Although often overlooked, handouts and print instructional materials continue to serve as useful tools. They are available at the Information/Reference Desk in a kiosk and in electronic form linked from the Hardin Web site, and selected ones are offered as inserts in the resource folders made available in the classes and workshops. Handouts are always a work in progress, as they are constantly re-evaluated and updated by the reference staff. When available, commercial materials are used, since the quality of the graphics is often better. Furthermore, if free, these handouts save the cost of copying, time, and use of human resources.

The open-enrollment, or skills workshops, provide hands-on opportunities for patrons to learn about new electronic resources and improve their database searching skills. Patrons preregister for these sessions, which last anywhere from one to two hours and are generally taught in the library's computerized classrooms in the Information Commons. A core set of classes has been offered on a regular basis, typically several times a semester. These workshops cover topics such as searching MEDLINE and PubMed, using Web of Science, and utilizing evidence-based medicine resources. From 1997 to 2002, Hardin offered a total of 589 instructional sessions, 338 of which were open-enrollment workshops.

In recent years, workshop attendance has been low. Although patrons often register for the classes, they frequently fail to attend. The first attempt to improve attendance was to drastically increase the promotion of the classes. Fliers were placed in buildings on campus, notices were sent to department mailing lists, and announcements were included in the hospital's daily newsletter. Initially, the response was positive. The number of people registering for the workshops increased and there was renewed excitement over the classes. However, despite increased registrations, attendance remains poor. Interestingly, the only classes that consistently draw large crowds are the sessions on using the EndNote bibliographic management software. This continues to be the primary workshop topic requested by patrons.

Along with the increased promotion of the workshops, an e-mail reminder is sent to each registrant a week prior to the sessions. Several years ago, a $5 fee was charged to patrons failing to attend a workshop. Some libraries have been known to charge a fee for attendance to compensate for the level of workload involved.[7] Despite these efforts, attendance continued to be a problem. It became clear that the existing workshop model did not make the best use of the librarians' time and energy. The decision was made to reduce the number of times each class is offered each semester to reach larger audiences.

Tailored workshops allow librarians to offer classes on any range of topics to groups and organizations requesting instruction. The content presented is geared to the information needs of the attendees and focuses on resources that would be of interest to them. Often the groups assembled consist of undergraduate or graduate students. Course instructors frequently require that their students participate in the session they have scheduled. Attendance is usually good, although the overall number of tailored workshops offered by Hardin Library is far fewer than the library would like to offer. Many groups do not know that this educational opportunity exists. The library director has met with success by contacting deans and department liaisons to promote these workshops. There is also the potential to reach out to the faculty across campus. Hardin Library now offers faculty development sessions several times each semester for those affiliated with the College of Medicine. The session content varies and attendance has been mixed. Faculty have offered positive feedback with the online evaluation form used at the completion of each session. Such programs will be offered to other colleges and departments on the health sciences campus in the future.

Walk-in consultations are handled by on-call staff between the hours of 2:00 p.m. and 3:00 p.m. daily on a rotational basis. This allows a staff member to be available for patrons needing some extra attention or guidance using either the online catalog or online databases. Due to the sporadic and unpredictable nature of walk-in consultations, sometimes the staff member scheduled for any given day is not available. Whenever possible, the librarians now promote scheduled consultations, as described next.

Scheduled reference consultations are arranged between library staff and individual patrons or small groups. Although librarians at Hardin have always performed these consultations, in recent years the sessions have increased in number. Reminiscent of the days of mediated searching, these one-on-one sessions yield very effective teaching opportunities, since the patron's specific area of interest is addressed. These consultations enable patrons to sit with a librarian to discuss their research interests. Librarians discuss which databases best meet a patron's needs and how to go about searching them. Librarians involved in the consultations continually find the patrons to be extremely thankful for the individual attention. It is not uncommon for the participants to continue to contact the librarian they have worked with for additional assistance as their research progresses. It has become clear to those librarians teaching classes and providing consultations that the consultations often offer patrons a much more valuable service. To learn to search MEDLINE with a group of people is one thing. To be guided through the process of searching MEDLINE on your specific topic of interest is quite another.

Course-integrated instruction has received increased attention at Hardin Library. These sessions may occur at the library or in the lecture classroom when the group of students is large. Ideally, the course instructor and librarian meet ahead of time to discuss what skills the students should take away from the session. If there is a relevant assignment, the librarian will try to incorporate it into the discussion and demonstration. The goal of these sessions is for students to strengthen their information literacy skills in the more meaningful context of their coursework. Hardin Library hopes to expand its course-integrated instruction in the future. In fall 2003, librarians partnered with the College of Pharmacy to teach first- and third-year pharmacy students in both lectures and hands-on laboratory sessions, scheduled throughout the semester. This cooperative effort totaled approximately thirty-seven contact hours for the librarians involved. There is great potential to collaborate with health sciences faculty to guide students in locating and evaluating quality resources and information.

Declining attendance at open-enrollment workshops has prompted the librarians at Hardin to put more responsibility on the participants themselves. The new focus is to encourage groups to plan times for librarians to come and present on any topic desired. Groups are encouraged to have librarians come to their particular clinic, lab, or classroom to give participants the chance to receive instruction on their own turf.[8] If the group is small enough, an overhead projector is not necessary. A few participants will sit around a computer and learn together in a more informal atmosphere. Whenever possible, instruction will focus on the specific research questions of the participants. In a sense, these sessions will function as a group reference consultation. By putting the responsibility for arranging the sessions on the patrons themselves, there is less chance that the participants will fail to attend.

In addition to the aforementioned educational programs, several cooperative projects will reach even more patrons. Hardin Library received a grant to expand the use of PDAs within the College of Pharmacy. The librarians have also been invited to partner with the College of Nursing to create Web-based tutorials focused on using the library's resources. Many other opportunities will present themselves as the librarians continue to strengthen their working relationships with faculty throughout the university.

EVALUATION METHODS

Several methods have been used to evaluate Hardin Library's education program, including the following:

- Publisher and vendor Web statistics are entered into a matrix for analysis of leased indexes and databases. Page counts for various Web pages on the Hardin site are tracked. These usage statistics are viewed for the selection of resources to be included in class offerings.
- Postclass survey instruments are linked to specific sessions and instructors (see Figure 6.1). These are used to evaluate the quality and organization of class content.
- When patrons ask questions or comment about the education program, librarians note the selection of resources, content of educational offerings, and publicity (or lack thereof).
- In spring 2003, the public services area of the Hardin Library conducted an anonymous survey in which the entire health science campus faculty, staff, and students were invited to participate. This was followed up by focus group sessions to gain valuable feedback on patron needs.
- Personal observation by the library staff regarding patrons' use of resources both before and after skills sessions, and one-on-one sessions, such as research consultations, provide opportunities to observe and enhance patrons' skill levels.
- The instructional services database report form is used to track the types of sessions that are conducted in a campus-wide library system. This information is used to detect levels of involvement or gaps on a campus-wide level for the various health science colleges.

CONCLUSION

Hardin Library has a renewed focus on and interest in education. The library has seen tremendous change in recent years and expects this trend to continue. Those involved in library instruction realize that the future of higher education is hard to predict. Although some may view this as a challenge, Hardin Library chooses to see this as an opportunity to continually reassess services and transform the methods used to teach patrons.

Workshop 0323 ▼	EndNote, May 21, 2003, Instructors: Denise Britgen, Nancy Murphy, Linda Roth ▼
College of Public Health ▼	Status: (check one) ⃝ Faculty ⃝ Staff ⃝ Student

I felt that the **instructor/presenter** was knowledgeable
⃝ **Strongly Agree** ⃝ **Agree** ⃝ **Neutral (N/A)** ⃝ **Disagree** ⃝ **Strongly Disagree**

I felt that the **instructor/presenter** was well prepared / organized
⃝ **Strongly Agree** ⃝ **Agree** ⃝ **Neutral (N/A)** ⃝ **Disagree** ⃝ **Strongly Disagree**

I felt that the **instructor/presenter** was an effective presenter
⃝ **Strongly Agree** ⃝ **Agree** ⃝ **Neutral (N/A)** ⃝ **Disagree** ⃝ **Strongly Disagree**

I felt that the **instructor/presenter** was responsive to questions
⃝ **Strongly Agree** ⃝ **Agree** ⃝ **Neutral (N/A)** ⃝ **Disagree** ⃝ **Strongly Disagree**

I learned **concepts** that will help me find information or conduct research
⃝ **Strongly Agree** ⃝ **Agree** ⃝ **Neutral (N/A)** ⃝ **Disagree** ⃝ **Strongly Disagree**

I was able to **practice** new skills in finding information or conducting research
⃝ **Strongly Agree** ⃝ **Agree** ⃝ **Neutral (N/A)** ⃝ **Disagree** ⃝ **Strongly Disagree**

Instructional materials were useful/relevant
⃝ **Strongly Agree** ⃝ **Agree** ⃝ **Neutral (N/A)** ⃝ **Disagree** ⃝ **Strongly Disagree**

The session was **well organized**
⃝ **Strongly Agree** ⃝ **Agree** ⃝ **Neutral (N/A)** ⃝ **Disagree** ⃝ **Strongly Disagree**

The **facility** was conducive to learning
⃝ **Strongly Agree** ⃝ **Agree** ⃝ **Neutral (N/A)** ⃝ **Disagree** ⃝ **Strongly Disagree**

Overall, I would give this session a grade of
⃝ A   ⃝ B   ⃝ C   ⃝ D   ⃝ F

What was the **most useful** part of this session?

What was the **least useful** part of this session?

What would you add to this session to make it more useful to other students?

Please submit your comments or clear all fields and start over
| Submit | Reset this form |

FIGURE 6.1. Hardin Library for the Health Sciences Class/Workshop Evaluation.

NOTES

1. *Fact Book 2003,* Office of University Relations, University of Iowa. Available: <http://www.uiowa.edu/%7Eour/fact.book/>.

2. Hardin Library for the Health Sciences, University of Iowa. Statistical Information on the Hardin Library for the Health Sciences. Available: <http://www.lib.uiowa.edu/hardin/libstats.html>.

3. McKibbon, K. Ann, Haynes, R. Brian, Walker Dilks, Cynthia J., Ramsden, Michael F., Ryan, Nancy C., Baker, Lynda; Flemming, Tom, and Fitzgerald, Dorothy. "How Good Are Clinical MEDLINE Searches? A Comparative Study of Clinical End-User and Librarian Searches." *Computers and Biomedical Research* 23 (1990):583-593.

4. Wildemuth, Barbara M. and Moore, Margaret E. "End-User Search Behaviors and Their Relationship to Search Effectiveness." *Bulletin of the Medical Library Association* 83(July 1995):294-304.

5. Bren, Barbara, Hilleman, Beth, and Topp, Victoria. "Effectiveness of Hands-On Instruction of Electronic Resources." *Research Strategies* 16(1998):41-51.

6. Hardin Library Strategic Planning Group. "Meeting Information Needs of the Health Professions at the University of Iowa," Iowa City: University of Iowa. March 1, 1995.

7. Sollenberger, Julia and Smith, Bernie T. "Teaching Computer Searching to Health Care Professionals: Why Does It Take So Long?" In *User Education in Health Sciences: A Reader,* edited by M. Sandra Wood. Binghamton, NY: The Haworth Press, 1995, 117-122.

8. Feldman, Jonquil D. and Kochi, Julia K. "Making Housecalls: An Alternative to Library Classroom Instruction." In *User Education in Health Sciences: A Reader,* edited by M. Sandra Wood. Binghamton, NY: The Haworth Press, 1995, 79-85.

NOTES

1. Available at TILT Group of University Relations, University of Iowa. Available: http://www.uiowa.edu/~tilt/index.html.

2. The University for the Health Sciences, University of Iowa. Historical Information on the Hardin Library for the Health Sciences. Available: http://www.uiowa.edu/hardin/history.

3. Meerbergen A., Ann, Thomas K. Bate, Walter Fisher, Susan J. Ramsden, Shepard H. K. and Nancy C. D. U. and others Bloomington, Lowe and Ferguson, Larry Lee, Brian Cocking Ann Oliver of MEDLINE Searches. "A Comparative Study of User-and End-User and Librarian Searches," Computers and Biomedical Research, 23 (1990): 583-593.

4. W. Walsch, Deborah M. and Nicora, Margaret T. "End-User Search Behaviors and Their Relationship to Search Effectiveness," Bulletin of the Medical Library Association 8 (July 1993): 296-304.

5. Brett Durrant, Hillmann, Beth, and Tipp, Skertson. "Effectiveness of Hands-On Instruction of Electronic Resources," Research Strategies, 16 (1998): 41-51.

6. Hardin Library Search Team Group. "Measuring Up," Measuring Use of the Hardin Information at the University of Iowa, Iowa City: University of Iowa, March 3, 1995.

7. Soifschutz, Julia and Smith, Sonia. "E-Teaching Computer Searching to Health Care Professionals: Some Ideas in Take Bookmarks" in Best Education in Libraries and Internet. A Primer edited by M. Mindel, Wade Bindfenster, NYC: The Alliance Press 1999: 113-123.

8. Fescinist, Joseph D. and Kessler, Jodi R. "Making Distance the Alternative to Library Research Instruction," in The Educator in Media Services. A Primer edited by M. Smith, Wood Binghamton, NY: The Haworth Press, 1998: 29-55.

Chapter 7

Medical Informatics Intervention: Teaching the Teaching Residents at Christiana Care Health System

Sharon Easterby-Gannett
Ellen M. Justice

SETTING

The Christiana Care Health System is a partnership of health care providers and hospitals based in Wilmington, Delaware. As one of the largest health care providers in the Mid-Atlantic Region, the system includes two clinical medical libraries and two consumer health libraries. Emergency medicine and internal medicine residents affiliated with the system's teaching hospitals attend Medical Morning Report (MMR) each day to discuss patients' cases. In conjunction with these meetings, third-year residents devote four weeks to a teaching rotation in which they research clinical questions and teach and direct discussion based on the cases presented.

Medical librarians have been attending MMR at this health system for over a decade. A library staff member who has attended MMR as a part of the clinical medical library program since 1998 noticed a change at these meetings beginning in 1999. Instead of turning to the clinical librarian to ask for a literature search, the chief resident would ask the teaching resident (TR) to conduct the search. When a

Thank you to all who helped make this chapter a reality. Special thanks to Hayim S. Weiss for guiding the development of the statistical information; Cynthia J. Clendenin for providing editing expertise; Barbara J. Henry for giving useful feedback; Margaret L. Crosson for tallying the data; and Christine C. Chastain-Warheit and Diane G. Wolf for their encouragement and support.

TR announced at MMR that no information was available on a drug except the information from the drug insert, the librarian decided to ask the attending physician, at the close of the session, how certain anyone can be about the information retrieval skills of the TRs. Her questions to the attending physician were: "When a TR is not finding any information, how do you know that there is no information to find?" and "Is anyone noting whether the TR is developing any information retrieval skills?" Following this discussion, the two clinical medical librarians who share attendance at MMR became involved in the TR block.

The librarians' role in the TR block has evolved into a Medical Informatics Intervention (MII), which entails an initial survey requesting information about the TR's familiarity with technology and information retrieval skills, baseline search, pre- and postinformatics rating scale, and approximately five hours of instruction during a four-week block. Twenty-four TRs have completed the MII since 2001. The intervention is an attempt to teach evidence-based medicine (EBM) searching skills and to develop the habit of seeking information based on rigorous science. According to the initial surveys completed by the TRs, only 48 percent have had training in medical database searching.

The need for an informatics intervention has been cited in the medical literature.[1-2] According to Masys, "[u]se of information technologies is an essential component of evidence-based medicine and needs to be woven throughout the fabric of . . . medical education."[1] Shortliffe defined medical informatics as "the rapidly developing scientific field that deals with . . . retrieval and optimal use of biomedical information, data, and knowledge for problem solving and decision-making."[3]

The TR block created by Internal Medicine and Emergency Medicine is loosely modeled after a block developed by Jefferson Medical College and is designed to refine the residents' ability to teach as well as to improve their retrieval of medical literature from computerized sources. Evidence in the literature supports the creation of such a block. One author concludes that "[e]mergency medicine residents have not had sufficient computer training prior to residency."[4] Another author says that "[d]espite the identification of several barriers to obtaining additional computer training, particularly lack of time and the high cost of computers, seventy-one percent of respondents believed computer training should be mandatory during residency."[5] For each block, a third-year resident is assigned the role of teaching resident. The TR is not included in the direct inpatient care schedule but acts as teacher and consultant to the teams of residents and medical students.

EDUCATIONAL APPROACHES

The medical librarians draft a general lesson plan for the four-week teaching block. The plan includes one-on-one training, informal discussions with the TR, recommendations of useful tutorials, and a discussion about integrating EBM searching techniques into newly acquired MEDLINE searching abilities. Because medical librarians attend MMR three times per week, the sessions with the TRs are usually held after the report session that the librarian attended. The TR and librarian focus on the clinical questions from MMR, and the librarian demonstrates the use of appropriate resources and effective searching techniques. Several means are used to track the progress of the TRs, including the general lesson plan and a list of skills to be covered, complemented by notes written in a journal format by the medical librarians.

To assess each TR's MEDLINE searching skills at the beginning of the MII, a baseline search is assigned to the resident. The resident is asked to spend about fifteen minutes formulating a search strategy, executing the search using Ovid MEDLINE, and selecting citations. After the search is completed, the TR is asked to print the search strategy and results and review them with the librarian. The librarian spends about fifteen minutes discussing the resident's strategy, pointing out strengths and demonstrating alternative search strategies. This interaction also gives the resident and librarian an opportunity to discuss the clinical reasoning used to formulate the strategy and select citations.

The medical librarians outline specific skills to be learned during their block. TRs rate themselves on thirteen specific skills. The results help the librarians customize the instruction to address the skills with the lowest ratings. The self-assessment is administered again at the end of the informatics intervention to determine whether the TRs perceive themselves as having improved specific skills.

The librarians share attendance at MMR so that each TR spends time with each librarian during their block. The primary method of instruction emphasizes important aspects of searching such as using MeSH (Medical Subject Headings) and formulating a clinical question based on the Patient, Intervention, Comparison, Outcome (PICO) model. The practice of working one-on-one encourages experiential learning and provides opportunities for the librarians and residents to discuss the following tasks:

- Formulating effective clinical questions
- Choosing appropriate databases
- Using effective searching techniques
- Selecting the best possible evidence from the search results

The librarians discuss and demonstrate appropriate searching techniques in a variety of databases including Ovid MEDLINE, Ovid Cochrane Database of Systematic Reviews, Journals@Ovid, MD Consult, MICROMEDEX, and the Natural Medicines Comprehensive Database. Printing full-text articles or information from databases is also highlighted. MEDLINE is primarily emphasized and detailed searching techniques are discussed. In teaching MD Consult, the emphasis is on demonstrating advanced searching techniques. In MICROMEDEX the drug monographs, clinical reviews, toxicology information, and drug interactions tool are highlighted. The Medical Libraries home page on the health care system Intranet is demonstrated for each of the TRs so they know the resources available and how to access them from anywhere in the hospital twenty-four hours a day.

After a librarian has demonstrated search techniques in each of the databases or library resources, the TR is given the opportunity to apply the techniques. The librarian guides the searches as needed by helping to define an appropriate clinical question and making suggestions to refine search strategies. The TR is encouraged to explain clinical aspects of the question to help focus the search. The librarian shares searching expertise and demonstrates effective techniques. Appropriate citations and full-text articles are printed. After reviewing the information, the TR conveys the clinical pearls to fellow residents either orally or in writing.

Individualized instruction is favored as it allows for a collaborative approach to locating the information needed to answer clinical questions that may influence patient care. The TRs economize efforts by spending their time with the librarian learning searching skills that can save time in the future and, simultaneously, using this opportunity to answer the clinical questions posed by their colleagues.

EVALUATION METHODS

Teaching MEDLINE search skills to the TRs is the foundation used to introduce varied techniques that can be applied in other medical databases. Once these skills are learned, it is easier to integrate EBM search strategies. The librarians keep notes to track what has been covered and also to discuss progress in teaching specific skills and databases. Tutorials such as MICROMEDEX, Introduction to Evidence-Based Medicine, and Ovid Tutorial are also recommended to the TRs but not required.

The MEDLINE Strategy Assessment Tool developed by a team at Duke University outlines some primary guides for effective searching.[6-7] Using some of the guides outlined by this tool, the baseline searches of twenty TRs were analyzed. According to the initial survey, although 68 percent of the TRs had used MEDLINE before the informatics intervention, only 55 percent divided a question into concepts, searched each concept separately, or combined sets correctly. Although 45 percent of TRs used MeSH terms whenever possible, the most appropriate heading was not used in every search strategy. Many strategies employed keywords combined with Boolean operators, thereby bypassing the Ovid MEDLINE mapping tool.

By primarily using keyword searching, the TR does not have the opportunity to use MeSH or apply subheadings. Only 45 percent used subheadings, but 70 percent did use appropriate limits such as publication date. According to Joanne G. Marshall,

> There is concern among librarians that end users may rely too heavily on the Text Word search capability even when appropriate MeSH terminology is available. End users may not know how to use MeSH or may not recognize the added value of using MeSH terms.[8]

The MII stresses the importance of using MeSH whenever possible. TRs are made aware that keyword searching can be fraught with pitfalls.

TRs use keyword searching as a primary search strategy in MD Consult and UpToDate because usually they can find something applicable. Responses to the initial survey indicate that virtually all of the TRs were comfortable using MD Consult at the beginning of the block. Some TRs state that one of the difficulties they have using MD Consult is a high retrieval rate with low precision, making it time-consuming to find relevant citations. MD Consult defaults to sorting search results by full-text first, so the first several citations may not be germane to the clinical question. TRs learn to change this default to display the most relevant citations first. The librarians also explain the use of bracket commands and truncation that can refine a search strategy.

To study the impact of the informatics intervention on specific skills related to clinical information retrieval, a weighted score-based system was used to analyze the results of the Informatics Rating Scale (see Appendix). Data are combined for three different TR groups covering the 2001 to 2003 academic years. A slightly different rating scale was used in the 2001-2002 academic year; therefore, the totals (N) are dissimilar for some of the rating scale statements. The score for applying advanced limits increased from 2.9 before the intervention (BI) to 4.6 after the intervention (AI), demonstrating a 59 percent improvement. The score for those saying they used subheadings increased from 2.5 BI to 4.5 AI, indicating an 80 percent improvement. TRs expressed a better comfort level with searching MEDLINE after they learned the search techniques, allowing them to focus on relevant studies. There was a 156 percent improvement in TRs stating that they know how to use bracket commands, an advanced searching technique, in MD Consult. The TRs searching Ovid's EBM databases realized a 126 percent improvement.

By teaching the TRs better searching techniques in various databases, librarians can help them save time as they search for information in support of patient care and research. The ability to search medical databases in a reasonable amount of time increased 45 percent, from 3.1 BI to 4.5 AI (see Appendix). Studies show that physicians' and residents' pursuit rates for finding answers to clinical questions that arise during patient encounters are 30 percent or lower.[9-10] Michael

L. Green and colleagues suggest that one possible explanation for low pursuit rates is reported time constraints.[9-11] It has also been reported that difficulty with strategies, question formation, and physical fatigue accounted for residents' major searching problems. Inpatient responsibilities, time, and access to the library are the reasons for their perceived barriers to retrieving articles.[6] These studies indicate that clinicians believe they do not have enough time to address patient-oriented clinical questions and to retrieve useful information.

FUTURE PLANS

In the future, EBM searching techniques will be incorporated earlier in the TR block. Ways to formulate EBM search strategies called "hedges" will also be introduced. A follow-up questionnaire will be given to the TRs six months after their graduation from residency to determine whether the intervention has long-term effects on search techniques and information-seeking behavior.

CONCLUSION

Bridging the gap between the clinical arena and the medical informatics realm is one of the difficulties in EBM. The MII is intended to help close the gap. One goal was to use this intervention to demonstrate to TRs that they can conduct a proper search quickly if they formulate a well-built clinical question, select the appropriate resources, and use effective searching techniques. The MII appears to be working. Based on the Informatics Rating Scale, observation, and discussion, TRs utilize more effective search techniques to find clinically relevant medical information in support of patient care. They also become more familiar with library resources during the teaching block, enabling them to choose the appropriate resource to answer their patient care questions. The interactions between the TRs and librarians strengthen their collaborative relationship toward finding germane clinical information for patient care.

In addition to the goal of enhanced searching skills by residents, other benefits derived from library participation include:

- an increase in requests for library services (unrelated to morning reports),
- continuing education for the librarians,
- awareness of trends in health care that support collection and resource development,
- opportunities for on-the-spot teaching,
- increased knowledge of the major diseases treated at the health center, and
- promoting the health care system (and library services) to prospective residents.[12]

TRs find clinically relevant and evidence-based information to support patient care decision making after the informatics intervention, save time by using more effective searching techniques, and become more familiar with the medical libraries' resources. These instructional interactions have strengthened the relationship between TRs and librarians.

APPENDIX: FINDINGS FROM THE TEACHING RESIDENT BLOCK: PRE- AND POSTINFORMATICS RATING SCALE

Weighted score = Sum total/sum volume
BI = Before intervention
AI = After intervention
N = Population

Statement #6: I know how to use Ovid's advanced limits (e.g., age groups, publication types, journal subsets).

Score	BI *n*	AI *n*	BI score (120 possible)	AI score (120 possible)	BI weighted score	AI weighted score
Strongly agree	8	16	40	80		
Somewhat agree	2	7	8	28		
Undecided	2	1	6	3		
Somewhat disagree	4	0	8	0		
Strongly disagree	8	0	8	0		
Total N	24	24	70	111	2.9	4.6[b] (59% improvement)

Statement #7: I know how to use subheadings in OVID to refine my search.

Score	BI *n*	AI *n*	BI Score (65 possible)	AI Score (65 possible)	BI weighted score	AI weighted score
Strongly agree	2	8	10	40		
Somewhat agree	2	4	8	16		
Undecided	2	1	6	3		
Somewhat disagree	2	0	4	0		
Strongly disagree	5	0	5	0		
Total N[a]	13	13	33	59	2.5	4.5[b] (79% improvement)

Statement #8: I know how to search Ovid's Evidence-Based Medicine databases (e.g., Cochrane database).

Score	BI *n*	AI *n*	BI score (120 possible)	AI score (120 possible)	BI weighted score	AI weighted score
Strongly agree	1	13	5	65		
Somewhat agree	3	8	12	32		
Undecided	1	1	3	3		
Somewhat disagree	7	2	14	4		
Strongly disagree	12	0	12	0		
Total N	24	24	46	104	1.9	4.3[b] (126% improvement)

Statement #9: When searching medical databases, I find answers to my clinical questions in a reasonable amount of time.

Score	BI *n*	AI *n*	BI score (120 possible)	AI score (120 possible)	BI weighted score	AI weighted score
Strongly agree	2	12	10	60		
Somewhat agree	14	11	56	44		
Undecided	3	1	9	3		
Somewhat disagree	5	0	10	0		
Strongly disagree	0	0	0	0		
Total N	24	24	75	107	3.1	4.5[b] (45% improvement)

Statement #13: I know how to use the bracket commands (e.g., [ti], to refine my searches in MD Consult).

Score	BI *n*	AI *n*	BI score (120 possible)	AI score (120 possible)	BI weighted score	AI weighted score
Strongly agree	1	10	5	50		
Somewhat agree	2	8	8	32		
Undecided	1	5	3	15		
Somewhat disagree	3	1	6	2		
Strongly disagree	17	0	17	0		
Total N	24	24	39	99	1.6	4.1[b] (156% improvement)

[a]Total (N) is lower because the above statement did not appear on the rating scale during 2001-2002 academic year.
[b]Weighted averages rounded for simplification, not analysis.

NOTES

1. Masys, Daniel R. "Advances in Information Technology: Implications for Medical Education." *Western Journal of Medicine* 168(May 1998):341-347.

2. Greenes, Robert A. and Shortliffe, Edward H. "Medical Informatics: An Emerging Academic Discipline and Institutional Priority." *JAMA* 263(February 23, 1990): 1114-1120.

3. Shortliffe, Edward H. "Medical Informatics Meets Medical Education." *JAMA* 273(April 5, 1995):1061,1064-1065.

4. Jwayyed, Sharhabeel, Park, Tammy K., Blanda, Michelle, Wilber, Scott T., Gerson, Lowell W., Meerbaum, Sharon O., and Beeson, Michael S. "Assessment of Emergency Medicine Residents' Computer Knowledge and Computer Skills: Time for an Upgrade?" *Academic Emergency Medicine* 9(February 2002):138-145.

5. Jerant, Anthony F. "Training Residents in Medical Informatics." *Family Medicine* 31(July/August 1999):465-472.

6. Cabell, Christopher H., Schardt, Connie, Sanders, Linda, Corey, G. Ralph, and Keitz, Sheri A. "Resident Utilization of Information Technology: A Randomized Trial of Clinical Question Formation." *Journal of General Internal Medicine* 16(December 2001):838-444.

7. Schardt, Connie, Cabell, Chris, and Keitz, Sheri. "Morning Report: MEDLINE Strategy Assessment Tool." Durham, NC: Duke University Medical Center, 1999. Available: <http://www.mclibrary.duke.edu/respub/guides/mrtool.html>.

8. Marshall, Joanne G. "End-User Training: Does It Make a Difference?" In *User Education in Health Sciences Libraries: A Reader,* edited by M. Sandra Wood. Binghamton, NY: The Haworth Press, 1995, 123-134.

9. Green, Michael L., Ciampi, Marc A., and Ellis, Peter J. "Residents' Medical Information Needs in Clinic: Are They Being Met?" *American Journal of Medicine* 109(August 15, 2000):218-223.

10. Covell, David G., Uman, Gwen C., and Manning, Phil R. "Information Needs in Office Practice: Are They Being Met?" *Annals of Internal Medicine* 103(October 1985):596-599.

11. Williamson, J.W., German, P.S., Weiss, R., Skinner, EA., and Bowes, F. "Health Science Information Management and Continuing Education of Physicians." *Annals of Internal Medicine* 110(January 15, 1989):151-160.

12. Wolf, Diane G., Chastain-Warheit, Christine C., Easterby-Gannett, Sharon, Chayes, Marion C., and Long, Brad A. "Hospital Librarianship in the United States: At the Crossroads." *Journal of the Medical Library Association* 90(January 2002): 38-44.

Chapter 8

The Librarian's Role As Information Technology Educator at the University of South Alabama

Justin Robertson

INTRODUCTION

The librarian's primary role has always been that of a teacher. Although other responsibilities remain integral to the profession—archivist, preservationist, bibliographer, indexer, and so on—the librarian's fundamental objective is one of educational empowerment. True librarianship should never content itself by merely showing a patron where to find information; it must also take the responsibility of instructing people how to find, access, and retrieve information for themselves. From papyrus scrolls to megalithic electronic databases, the specific methods and tools may have changed significantly, but the overarching purpose remains constant: lead one's patrons to needed information, but show them the path on the way there.

Much has changed in academic libraries over the past two decades. The stalwart card catalog is gone, replaced by a computer with a complex and frequently bewildering online catalog. The familiar print subject index is rapidly being supplanted by its electronic counterpart, while many academic journals are finding their way online, complementing (if not always wholly replacing) their paper counterparts. Even the contents of entire books are becoming available electronically. Beyond these drastic changes found in customary library tools, a plethora of new information-related technology has altered the way people access, use, and organize information. Such tools include popular spreadsheet, presentation, and publishing software, and several new devices developed to keep information readily at hand.

It is within this realm of "nontraditional" information tools that the modern librarian needs to respond more proactively. Beyond simply demonstrating how to fulfill information needs—even beyond the route of traditional bibliographic instruction principles—librarians must educate users about using new technologies to access traditional information resources. Twenty years ago, the conscientious librarian would not have pointed new users to the card catalog and expected them to locate their own information. Instead, the librarian would have explained how to best utilize the card catalog and perhaps shown patrons how to use relevant print indexes. Furthermore, the librarian might have shown patrons where to find materials in the stacks and how to organize their information most effectively. It appears that some bibliographic instruction programs have forgotten these basic principles. The programs may demonstrate where, and even how, to find the best materials, but rarely deal with issues of utilizing and manipulating the information once it is found. Even though the tools have changed and become more complex, new concepts need to be incorporated into traditional bibliographic instruction programs.

SETTING

The University of South Alabama, part of the state's higher education school system, is located in Mobile on the state's Gulf Coast. The university's average enrollment is 12,000, with approximately 250 students enrolled in the College of Medicine program. The Biomedical Library itself is composed of three branches: the campus site, Medical Center site, and Children and Women's Hospital site. Each location caters to a particular audience, with the campus site focusing primarily on the academic needs of the biomedical students. The library as a whole boasts a large collection of online databases and full-text journals available to all university students.

EDUCATIONAL APPROACHES

Formal bibliographic instruction has always been a priority for Baugh Biomedical Library faculty. The majority of the library's professionals have been, at one time or another, actively involved in some aspect of library education. Different bibliographic instruction

(BI) sessions are designed to cover a wide range of the university population, from students to faculty to support staff. BI sessions can range from one-on-one instruction to groups of sixty or more. In addition, these classes take on a variety of formats designed specifically for the particular needs or previous experience of patrons.

Two special BI sessions have been embedded in both College of Medicine and College of Allied Health courses each year. These sessions include a general overview lecture followed by a series of small-group follow-up classes. Students must complete and return library worksheets to the BI teacher, who in turn reports the results to the course instructor. Still, despite this diversity of bibliographic instruction sessions, the Biomedical Library had never created its own stand-alone, for-credit course. When the opportunity finally presented itself, the library eagerly embraced this new challenge that would enhance its educational responsibilities.

For several years, an elective called *Information Technology in Medicine* (designated as FMP 479) was taught under the auspices of the College of Medicine's Family Practice Department. This course concentrated on computer hardware, software, and the Internet, and featured classes on basic computer hardware and emerging technologies such as handheld computers. In addition, various popular software packages such as Word, PowerPoint, Access, Excel, and others were covered. The class was limited to ten students, with only one session of this month-long course concentrating on traditional medical informatics. During summer 2000 the course instructor left the University of South Alabama for another position. Rather than let the class languish, the Biomedical Library's director and the education coordinator arranged a meeting with the dean of the Family Practice department. They offered to assume responsibility for the class, positing that new physicians should be aware of the information technology available to them once they started practicing. The dean agreed and in the fall and winter of 2001 the librarians convened and began working on the next class session scheduled for April 2002.

The librarians decided to customize an existing class that would dovetail traditional research methodology with an examination of the evolving world of information technology. *Information Technology in Medicine* is taught as a for-credit, fourth-year elective for the university's medical students.

The first task was to create a revised syllabus (see Appendix A) that reflected the librarians' specific educational goals. Because the class met Monday through Thursday for four weeks, it was broken down into sixteen separate classes, with a wrap-up/question and answer session for the final (seventeenth) meeting. Using the existing syllabus as a framework, the course was rebuilt to meet new goals and specifications. Some material was revised, some new content was added, and in some instances, entire topics were removed due to either time considerations and/or perceived relevancy. Material added to the course was chosen primarily to help prepare physicians for the information technology they would face once they began practicing. Biweekly meetings were established and each librarian involved with the course was urged to attend. The library's education coordinator led the meetings, but contributions from all participants were encouraged. Planning began with a few major bedrock decisions upon which the rest of the class would be built.

The first such decision required that each participating librarian be responsible for at least one class session. Whenever possible, instructors were matched to the topics with which they had the most familiarity. Remaining sessions were matched according to interest, and in some cases the instructors had to learn more about their given topic before they felt prepared to teach it. It was also decided that although one instructor would lead each session, there would also be a backup or co-instructor. The rationale behind this decision was threefold. It ensured that students would receive additional attention as needed; it guaranteed that the co-instructor could step in as an "understudy" if the principal teacher was unavailable; and it meant that the librarians could share the heavy workload they would likely encounter when putting together particular sessions.

The next challenge involved providing cohesion to a class in which the instructors often changed from day to day. Constructing the course contents from the ground up—thematically, like a pyramid—seemed to solve this problem. Practically speaking, initial classes would discuss the most basic information, and each successive session would ideally build upon the one before it. Thus, the first session involved basic computer hardware, the second an overview of the Windows platform, and the next two sessions were dedicated to Windows and so forth, until the final class session had the students building their own simple Web pages. The hope was that as student knowledge and confidence grew, so would the complexity of each assignment, with tasks often depending upon information from a prior session. For example, the Web page exercise required that students use graphics created in an earlier session. This would also provide structure to a class that covered a range of material and was taught by many instructors.

The next consideration was how to accurately measure the varying skill levels students would bring to the class. Discussions with the previous class instructor revealed that all degrees of expertise—from intimidated novice to proficient user—should be anticipated; the trick was figuring out who knew what and how much before the class actually began. The previous instructor had created a basic computer skills survey that was handed out at the beginning of the first session. An identical questionnaire was given out on the last day to gauge the overall effectiveness of the class. The librarians emulated this approach, adapting the new questionnaire to reflect more accurately changes made in the course curriculum (see Appendix B).

As the instructors developed their particular sessions the biweekly meetings continued as forums for progress reports serving as "road tests" and highlighting each session's strengths and potential weaknesses. The form and content of individual sessions was not dictated by any standard formula or rigid structure. Aside from the fact that each class would conclude with an assignment, sessions were purposely constructed to serve the material being taught and the given instructor's teaching predilections. See <http://southmed.usouthal.edu/library/ref/fmp479/infoclass910.htm> for a detailed example of the Excel session, including presentations, relevant links, assignments, and other pertinent data. Some subjects, such as personal digital assistants (PDAs) and the overview of medical office software, consisted mostly of lectures and slide presentations, while other sessions such as graphics and Web design used live examples and dynamic interactions among the class participants and the instructor. Considerations were also given to class length. Scheduled to meet from 9:00 a.m. to noon with a lunch break and hands-on lab time afterward, many sessions simply did not warrant three hours of instruction. Even though classes frequently ended earlier, students were still expected to return and do their work in the afternoon. During this time, that day's instructors were required to be available to assist students as needed, a practice that is not unlike professors keeping specific office hours. Daily evaluation sheets were created. All of these were identical and given out at the end of each session, to gather student feedback regarding class content and instructor performance for each class.

The instructors wanted to ensure that the *Information in Technology* class developed a robust Web presence. The education coordinator built a Web site that would contain an overview of the class and archived materials from each session. All class handouts, PowerPoint presentation, tutorials, assignments, relevant links, and so on, are accessible online. Although this process was a time-intensive undertaking, the students found it quite helpful, particularly if they missed a class or misplaced a session's particular materials.

Particular products and platforms covered in specific sessions were considered for pragmatic reasons alone. PCs with Windows operating systems were discussed rather than Apple products. The software products covered (such as Word, PowerPoint, and Excel) were chosen because they are the most commonly used software packages. No assumptions were made on what students may encounter or prefer in the future; these decisions were made pragmatically.

Classes dealing with technological resources available from different vendors depended upon instructor judgment, product availability, and product cost. The PDA session, for example, examined a wide variety of the products currently available. Similarly, rather than introducing students to a single (and quite possibly expensive) Web editor, they were taught to code HTML by hand using Netscape Composer, a freely available authoring program. The burden of keeping class materials as relevant as possible depends on the instructors themselves. As new resources become available and others obsolete, session materials must be diligently monitored and updated. With the basic parameters set, instructors began finalizing the details of their particular sessions. A course overview, outlining what was covered during each session, can be found in the finalized syllabus (see Appendix A). More detailed information is available on the class Web site, <http://southmed.usouthal.edu/library/ref/fmp479/index. html>.

It should be noted that the final session serves as a general wrap-up in which students submit their final assignments and ask questions about any of the previous classes. During this session, two evaluation sheets are given to the students. One evaluation is identical to the computer skills questionnaire given out during the first session, while the other is intended to solicit student opinions, comments, and suggestions about the class as a whole. The education coordinator is designated to receive and keep all class documents, including assignments, questionnaires, and evaluations, and is responsible for grading all the assignments on a pass/fail basis. Grades are submitted to the university's Department of Medical Information for final processing.

Changes made to the course since its original incarnation reflect how professional librarians view current information technology issues in the world of medicine. Products that seemed relatively marginal to a doctor's future career such as Access and Publisher software were dropped from the syllabus to extend time spent on the Internet and medical informatics. Front Page, an HTML editing program, and information about voice input technology were also dropped. Overall, the new syllabus retained roughly 50 percent of the original class while the other half underwent serious revision. This compromise accurately reflected the librarians' goal to interject increased technological awareness into the traditional bibliographic instruction forum. At the same time, the class was also designed to provide in-depth instruction on research strategies and techniques. With these two separate, but related, goals in mind, the library taught the first *Information Technology in Medicine* class in April 2002.

As with many new ventures, everything looked simpler in black and white. Although the course was thoroughly planned in advance, when the sessions actually began, so did the real test of the librarians' planning abilities. It was immediately evident that several sessions needed to be shortened. For example, dedicating a class each to computer hardware and Windows proved to be too much, and in future classes these two topics were combined into a single session. This decision freed up an extra day for Web page development, which turned out to be extremely popular. Several students recommended that in the future it should be a two-day session. Other student comments, as well as instructor observation, offered further insight into how the class could be improved upon. The course remains a work in progress.

EVALUATION METHODS

The information gleaned from the exit surveys and session commentaries, on the whole, proved to be positive. The students reacted favorably to the combination of technical information and medical informatics instruction, agreeing that it would be helpful in their professional lives. Although further fine-tuning is needed, the class remains on the College of Medicine's academic schedule.

Because this class has been taught only once, it would be unreliable to base success on any numerical data received from the identical sets of *Computer Skills* evaluation sheets handed out on the first and last days of class. Comparing the returned evaluations revealed that even the most technically savvy students found the class beneficial, while those who originally rated themselves as novice users boosted both their technical know-how and, perhaps more significantly, their computer self-confidence.

CONCLUSION

By and large, the instructors found this experience rewarding. The general consensus was that the class forged new and positive traditions for bibliographic instruction at Baugh Biomedical Library. Librarians attained credibility as teachers. The BI department helped traditional medical informatics meet emerging information technology. Although it will take a great deal of work to keep this initiative going, it is essential to the continued relevancy of the modern library professional.

APPENDIX A:
COLLEGE OF MEDICINE ELECTIVE FMP 479

Information Technology in Medicine Syllabus
Spring 2002
<http://southmed.usouthal.edu/library/ref/fmp479/>

Course Description:	By the end of this course students will have been exposed to a variety of resources and tools applicable to information technology useful during continuing medical education and future practice.
Course Schedule:	March 11 through April 4 (Mondays thru Thursdays) and Friday April 5, 2002—**Class:** 9:00 a.m., **Lab:** 1:00 p.m.
Course Directors:	Justin Robertson and Tom Williams
Session Instructors:	Judy Burnham, Jie Li, Sally Murray, Justin Robertson, Ellen Sayed, Jana Slay, Geneva Staggs, Diane Williams and Tom Williams
Course Particulars/ Requirements:	**Office Hours:** An instructor will be available the rest of day of instruction. **Text:** Each instructor has provided reading material. **Assignments:** Each assignment should be clearly labeled, saved, and submitted by the due date. Missing or incomplete assignments will be factored into the determinations of final grades. **Computers:** All the necessary software for assignments is available in the COM computer lab on the second floor of CMB Biomedical Library. **Attendance:** All students are expected to attend class. You will be responsible for all materials and announcements made during class, whether or not you are present. **Grades:** Pass/Fail based on attendance, participation, and assignments. **Disabilities:** In accordance with the Americans with Disabilities Act, students with bona fide disabilities will be afforded reasonable accommodation. The Office of Special Student Services will certify a disability and advise faculty members of reasonable accommodations. If you have a specific disability that qualifies you for academic accommodations, please notify Justin Robertson, and provide certification from Disability Services (Office of Special Student Services). The Office of Special Student Services is directed by Ms. Bernita Pulmas and is located in the student center, Room 270, phone 460-7212. **Changes:** Policies and/or requirements specified in this syllabus are subject to modification as circumstances dictate. If any changes are necessary, they will be communicated in writing to the students.

Class Session Schedule

March 11	Class 1: Computer Hardware—Tom Williams/Sally Murray
March 12	Class 2: Windows 95-98—Judy Burnham/Geneva Staggs
March 13	Class 3: Microsoft Word (part 1)—Jana Slay/Diane Williams
March 14	Class 4: Microsoft Word (part 2)—Jana Slay/Diane Williams
March 18	Class 5: Internet (part 1)—Sally Murray/Justin Robertson
March 19	Class 6: Internet (part 2)—Sally Murray/Justin Robertson
March 20	Class 7: Graphics—Sally Murray/Justin Robertson
March 21	Class 8: PowerPoint—Justin Robertson/Sally Murray
March 25	Class 9: Microsoft Excel (part 1)—Ellen Sayed/Diane Williams
March 26	Class 10: Microsoft Excel (part 2)—Ellen Sayed/Diane Williams
March 27	Class 11: Online Medical References (part 1)—Justin Robertson/Sally Murray/Geneva Staggs
March 28	Class 12: Online Medical References (part 2)—Justin Robertson/Sally Murray/Geneva Staggs
April 1	Class 13: Medical Office Software—Jie Li/Justin Robertson
April 2	Class 14: Handheld Computing—Jie Li/Justin Robertson
April 3	Class 15: CME—Judy Burnham/Tom Williams
April 4	Class 16: Creating Web Pages—Sally Murray/Justin Robertson
April 5	Class 17: Wrap-Up—Justin Robertson/Sally Murray

APPENDIX B: BASIC PERSONAL COMPUTER
CONFIDENCE SURVEY (BBL 479)

Circle either YES or NO	Knowledge/Skill
Hardware	
YES NO	In shopping for a computer, I would know what processor, speed, memory, hard drive, printer, and monitor I want.
YES NO	I would feel comfortable taking a new computer and printer out of the boxes and setting them up.
Keyboard	
YES NO	I can type comfortably without looking at my hands at a reasonable speed.
YES NO	I feel comfortable using a mouse to run programs, highlight text, and select menu items.
Software—General	
YES NO	I know what system software such as Windows does.
YES NO	I know the uses of word processing software and can name a word processing software package.
YES NO	I know the uses of spreadsheet software and can name a spreadsheet software package.
YES NO	I know the uses of presentation and graphics software and can name an example software package.
YES NO	I understand the purpose of a Web browser and can name one.
Systems Software—GUI Interfaces	
YES NO	I can buy a new software package and install it on a computer.
YES NO	I can remove a program from my hard drive and delete it from the program list.
YES NO	I can organize my files into folders and find a file I need to open or move.
YES NO	I can store files on floppy disks or on the hard drive and move them back and forth.
YES NO	I can control my display colors, background, and resolution, and set the time and date.
YES NO	I can run several programs at once, going from one to the other.
YES NO	I know how to properly shut down a computer, or restart it without killing the power.

Word Processing Software		
YES	NO	I can create, save, and print a new word processing document.
YES	NO	I can find and open an old document, edit it, and print it out.
YES	NO	I can format the text in the document using different fonts, font sizes, bold, italics, and underline.
YES	NO	I can align paragraphs to be left, centered, right, or justified.
YES	NO	I can create bulleted lists or numbered lists.
YES	NO	I can cut, copy, and paste words, sentences, or paragraphs.
YES	NO	I can set margins and page orientation (portrait or landscape).
YES	NO	I can add headers and footers to include page numbers.
YES	NO	I can create tables in a word processing document.
Spreadsheets		
YES	NO	I can create, save, and print a new spreadsheet document that does calculations.
YES	NO	I understand cell addresses.
YES	NO	I can format a number in a cell to be currency, percent or a number with a particular number of decimal places.
YES	NO	I can change the width and height of cells.
YES	NO	I can write a formula that will add a row of cells in a spreadsheet.
YES	NO	I can write a formula that will use functions such as AVERAGE in a spreadsheet.
YES	NO	I can add borders and shading to cells in a spreadsheet.
YES	NO	I can create a chart or graph from a spreadsheet using spreadsheet software.
Presentation Software		
YES	NO	I can create a slide using presentation software.
YES	NO	I can create an entire slide presentation using presentation software.
YES	NO	I can add transitions to the slides.
YES	NO	I can add build effects or animation to the bulleted lists in a slide presentation.
YES	NO	I can draw geometric figures such as organization charts with a graphics or paint program.
YES	NO	I can use design templates to make the slides colorful.
YES	NO	I can print out slides or handouts using presentation software.
YES	NO	I can use data projection equipment to present my slide presentation from a computer.

Graphics	
YES NO	I understand that there are different file formats for graphics files which determine the number of colors that can be used and the resolution of the image.
YES NO	I can crop and resize the image.
YES NO	I can add graphics (pictures or clip art) to a word processing document or slide presentation.
YES NO	I can adjust the color, brightness, and contrast of the image.
E-Mail	
YES NO	I feel comfortable using e-mail software.
YES NO	Given a friend's e-mail address, I can send a message.
YES NO	I can read and reply to an e-mail message.
YES NO	I can forward an e-mail message to other addresses.
YES NO	I can save an e-mail message into a folder that I have created.
YES NO	I can attach files to e-mail messages.
YES NO	I can check my e-mail from a remote location using a different computer from my own.
WWW/Browsers	
YES NO	I can use a Web browser such as Netscape to access the World Wide Web.
YES NO	I can use a Web search engine such as Infoseek or Yahoo to find information on the Web.
YES NO	I can open a Web site from the address (www.dell.com) that I have seen in a magazine or on TV.
YES NO	I can set and edit bookmarks/favorites of my favorite Web sites.
YES NO	I can capture pictures from Web pages and save them.
YES NO	I can keep up with all of my user IDs and passwords for all my accounts.
YES NO	I can do a MEDLINE search.
YES NO	I feel comfortable using computer-based educational packages.
YES NO	I feel comfortable using computer-based textbooks and full-text journals such as SAM-CD or the PDR.

Name _____

Comments—What specific skills would you like to learn in this class?

Chapter 9

Using Computer-Based Case Studies for Developing Information Searching Skills and Implementing Evidence-Based Medicine at Jefferson Medical College

Anthony J. Frisby
Daniel G. Kipnis

INTRODUCTION

Since 1987, over 1,300 first-year medical students at Jefferson Medical College in Philadelphia, Pennsylvania, have completed a required medical informatics course. This course is the responsibility of the Scott Memorial Library's Education Services division. Designed to develop information searching skills and teach methods for evaluating evidence-based medicine, the course employs a combination of self-paced online tutorials and case studies. The case studies in particular have proven to be a very effective learning tool. Course evaluations are consistently positive, with comments citing the interesting case studies and the effectiveness and appropriateness of the teaching methods. This chapter describes the case development process, presents learner support issues for library staff, reviews the evaluation process and results, and identifies Jefferson's future plans for teaching successful information searching skills.

The authors thank Elizabeth G. Mikita, MLS, for her feedback and editing assistance in writing this chapter.

SETTING

Founded in 1824, Jefferson Medical College, one of the largest private medical schools in the United States, has more living graduates than any other medical school in the nation. The academic medical center includes Jefferson Medical College, Jefferson College of Health Professions, Jefferson College of Graduate Studies, and Thomas Jefferson University Hospitals, a 900-bed teaching facility. Scott Memorial Library serves the three colleges in the university and also functions as the library for the hospitals. *Medical Informatics* (IDEPT 123) is a required course for all first-year medical students. Over the past fifteen years, Education Services has experimented with a number of different methods for delivering the course content and developed this model to meet the current needs of Jefferson's students.

EDUCATIONAL APPROACHES

"Medical Informatics" began in 1989 as a live lecture to the entire 230-student class and followed with small-group sessions that included direct demonstrations of the databases and short practice exercises. Each session included nine to ten students, with some reshuffling if students missed sessions and needed to reschedule. This format was not very effective for the teaching staff or the students. The isolated exposure did allow students to become familiar with the library's information systems and to perform the required exercises, but since it was separate from any real context students could relate to, any learned skills were probably quickly forgotten. This approach did not reinforce the skills needed to be lifelong learners, a university goal for students.

To make instruction more efficient and relevant, Education Services librarians and instructional designers partnered with clinical faculty to develop realistic case studies. The first case includes considerable in-context support, or instructional scaffolding, that provides guidance on how to structure search questions and where it is appropriate to search for answers. Students can compare their questions, search parameters, and results with those developed by librarians. In later cases, this scaffolding is removed, which encourages students to recall and apply their new skills.

Table 9.1 shows the instructional design process followed in the development of the cases and screen captures of the final case studies as presented to the students. The lead instructional designer had been using Gagne's instructional design model for several years in the development of computer-based learning materials,[1-2] and that model was used for the tutorials and case studies in *Medical Informatics*.

TABLE 9.1. Gagne's instructional events.

Instructional event	Example
1. Gain attention	Identify start of module (opening screen, may include sound and animation)
2. Inform learners of objectives	List learning goals and why these are important to the learner (source of goals and how the learner will apply these goals in clinical practice)
3. Stimulate recall of prior learning	Provide an example learner is likely to already be familiar with (relate the new learning materials to something the learner is already familiar with, providing a foundation to build on)
4. Present the content	Begin actual tutorial or case study (the main body of the instructional content)
5. Provide learning guidance	Support instruction with examples and explanations (provide different examples that will appeal to different learners and learning styles)
6. Elicit performance	Allow learner to apply new knowledge or skills (allow the learner to use new knowledge and skills in solving new problems)
7. Provide feedback	Give appropriate feedback to learner's performance (provide detailed, corrective feedback, relate to objectives and real-world application)
8. Assess performance	Provide learner opportunity to perform again and evaluate that performance (usually the final, evaluated performance that counts toward the course grade)
9. Enhance retention and transfer	Review what knowledge and skills were presented and provide additional discussion of how this knowledge or skill works in real-world applications

Adapted from Gagne, R. M. and Driscoll, M. P. *Essentials of Learning for Instruction,* Second Edition. Englewood Cliffs, NJ: Prentice-Hall, 1988, 159.

Before beginning any instructional activity, it is important to first determine the instructional goals and identify certain characteristics about the learner. Jefferson's specific goals for this course are featured in Box 9.1. These goals are based on the Association of American Medical Colleges (AAMC) *Learning Objectives for Medical Student Education: Guidelines for Medical Schools,*[3] the American Library Association *Nine Information Literacy Standards for Student Learning,*[4] and Jefferson Medical College's *Learning Objectives for Medical Student Education.*

New Student Computing Survey

Each year a survey designed to measure prior computer use and computer-based learning experience is distributed to all first-year medical students. The results of this survey are beneficial in helping the library and Learning Resources Centers (campus computer labs) prepare for the new students. Interestingly, survey data indicate the often inappropriate reliance on general search engines to locate information relevant to health care, rather than the use of MEDLINE and evidence-based medicine databases. Sample survey questions and the responses received are featured in Box 9.2.

The first three instructional events (attention, objectives, prior recall) begin during the two-hour mandatory orientation session in the auditorium. This session:

- presents and discusses origination of course objectives, and explains why they are important to attendees as both students and clinicians;
- asks the students questions about their previous use of the medical information resources, specifically, how they accessed them and their purpose in using them; and
- demonstrates how to access the course materials and provides a short orientation to the resources needed to complete the case studies.

The remaining course requirements are entirely self-paced, computer-based instruction, including a pre-test to measure entering knowledge and skill level, two case studies, a post-test to demonstrate mastery of the objectives, and the course evaluation. Although only one lecture is required, optional hands-on assistance is provided at

BOX 9.1. Medical Informatics Course Objectives

Goal **The student will demonstrate an understanding of the need to engage in lifelong learning to stay abreast of relevant scientific advances.**

Behavioral Objectives
1. Recognize the need for additional information.
2. Identify relevant information resources including:
   - Colleagues and mentors
   - Librarians
   - Scott Memorial Library catalog (THOMCAT)
   - Electronic databases
   - Internet search engines
3. Request the services of an information professional when appropriate, i.e., reference librarian.
4. Use EBM resources and pharmacological databases to assess therapeutic interventions.

Goal **The student will demonstrate the ability to retrieve (from electronic databases and other resources), manage, and utilize biomedical information for solving problems and making decisions that are relevant to the care of individuals and populations.**

Behavioral Objectives
1. Formulate a search strategy to resolve clinical problem/question.
2. Select the appropriate information resource based on:
   - Content
   - Time frame
   - Depth
   - Authority
3. Define "Medical Subject Headings" (MeSH).
4. Briefly describe the indexing process of journal articles utilizing MeSH terms.
5. Describe the process of mapping.
6. Conduct an efficient and effective search using available tools including:
   - Keywords, authors, titles, controlled vocabularies
   - Boolean operators: and, or, not
   - Special commands: truncate, explode, focus, limits
   - Contrast the two MEDLINE electronic journal database interfaces, Ovid and PubMed.
7. Prescribe therapeutic intervention using evidence-based medical resources and pharmacological databases.

(continued)

(continued)

Goal	**The student will demonstrate the ability to critically evaluate the medical literature and to seek opportunities to expand understanding and appreciation of scientific discoveries and their applications.**
Behavioral Objectives	1. Evaluate the merit of retrieved information using the criteria of: • Content • Time frame • Depth • Authority 2. The ability to effectively teach patients and colleagues. • Obtain patient education materials and resources that are age and language appropriate. • Create educational sessions using presentation software to display text and graphics.

---

dedicated computer classroom support sessions offered several times during the three-week course. During these sessions, librarians from the education services and information services departments provide one-on-one coaching for students wanting the extra attention.

Instructional Event

Gain the Learner's Attention

Students complete a number of different online activities, including checking e-mail, participating in online group discussions, working with other online course materials, and general Web surfing. It is important to provide some way to identify the start of a new activity and get the learner in the right frame of mind for that structured learning activity. Once logged into the course Web site, students select the *Assignments* folder, and then select the pre-test or case studies. The pre-test is required, but the results are not included in any evaluation of the course. It provides both the library and the students with information about their entering knowledge and skill levels. Later it provides a starting-point score to compare with the post-test score. Pre-test scores consistently average in the upper sixties to low seventies on a scale of zero to 100. The pre-test and post-test questions come

BOX 9.2. Sample Questions and Responses from Jefferson Medical College Freshman Computing Survey

How many courses in your undergraduate program required you to use a computer?	Response (%)
No courses	6.53
1 course	7.53
2 courses	10.05
3 or more courses	74.87
Unanswered	1.00

Rate how confident you are that you could locate an authoritative discussion of a medical, pharmaceutical, or therapeutic topic on the Internet.	Response (%)
Extremely confident	22.11
Confident	45.22
Somewhat confident	25.12
Not at all	6.03
Unanswered	1.50

Rate how confident you are that you could locate an article using a bibliographic database such as MEDLINE or CINAHL.	Response (%)
Extremely confident	21.60
Confident	43.21
Somewhat confident	23.61
Not at all	10.05
Unanswered	1.50

Do you know what MeSH means?	Response (%)
Yes	58.79
No	39.69
Unanswered	1.50

Identify how important you think medical informatics skills will be to you as a physician.	Response (%)
Very important	69.34
Somewhat important	28.64
Not very important	1.00
Not at all important	0.0
Unanswered	1.00

from a pool of questions that are presented in a randomized structure by the university's course management system (Blackboard).

Figures 9.1-9.4 illustrate screens encountered by students using Blackboard to access "Medical Informatics" content. The first case study begins with a screen (Figure 9.1) identifying the resources this case will use, welcomes students, and introduces them to the activity they are about to begin. The next screen (Figure 9.2) introduces the clinical expert and begins to describe the patient scenario. As shown in Figure 9.3, the student "meets" the virtual clinician and a Socratic dialogue begins. As students progress through the case, standardized feedback (Figure 9.4) is presented when a response is submitted.

Inform the Learner of the Objectives

As noted, the course objectives are presented at the single orientation lecture for the course. In addition, upon entering the case studies students are presented with the purpose of the clinical visit and their responsibility in caring for the patient is established. Knowledge and skill acquisition is embedded in the case study to provide a realistic context for learning the content. Adult learning theories emphasize the importance of context as situated cognition,[5] meaning that skills

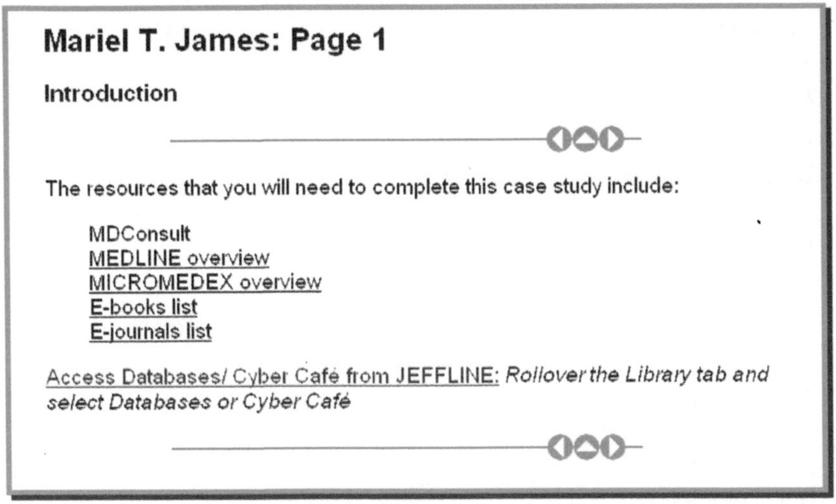

Mariel T. James: Page 1

Introduction

———————————————————————————————————◀❐▶-

The resources that you will need to complete this case study include:

    MDConsult
    MEDLINE overview
    MICROMEDEX overview
    E-books list
    E-journals list

Access Databases/ Cyber Café from JEFFLINE: *Rollover the Library tab and select Databases or Cyber Café*

———————————————————————————————————◀❐▶-

FIGURE 9.1. Introductory screen.

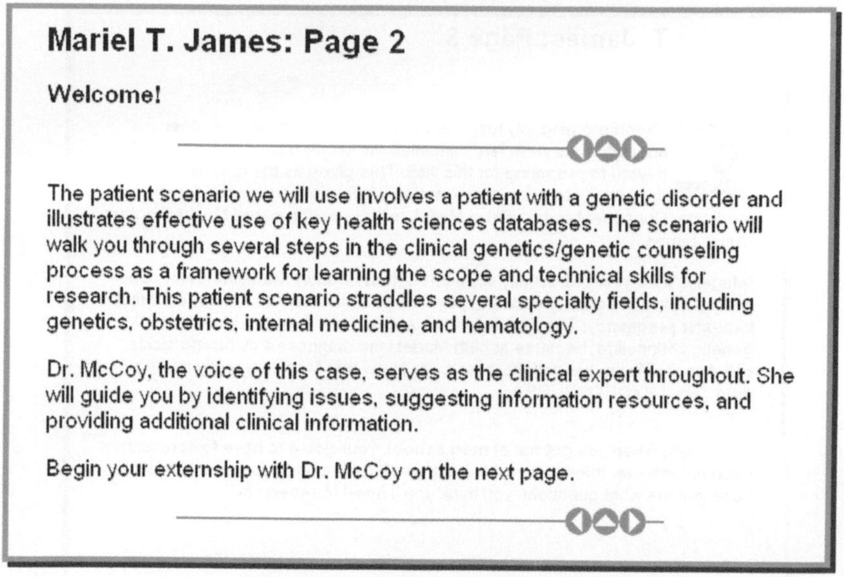

Mariel T. James: Page 2

Welcome!

The patient scenario we will use involves a patient with a genetic disorder and illustrates effective use of key health sciences databases. The scenario will walk you through several steps in the clinical genetics/genetic counseling process as a framework for learning the scope and technical skills for research. This patient scenario straddles several specialty fields, including genetics, obstetrics, internal medicine, and hematology.

Dr. McCoy, the voice of this case, serves as the clinical expert throughout. She will guide you by identifying issues, suggesting information resources, and providing additional clinical information.

Begin your externship with Dr. McCoy on the next page.

FIGURE 9.2. Patient scenario.

are best acquired in a setting as similar to their future application as possible. This transfer issue is reflected in the key problem of students doing well on multiple-choice exams, but being unable to actually apply the knowledge when out in the real world.

Case studies were selected as the instructional conduit for presenting the information literacy skills in this course. To develop realistic case studies, education services partnered with physicians in Jefferson's Family Medicine Department. The clinical partners were asked to think of common patient scenarios encountered by new students in the clinics and to walk the librarians through typical clinical encounters.

The cases were built using hypertext markup language (HTML) and custom scripts to record the students' progress and responses in an Oracle database. The custom development permitted the cases to be presented as a natural story, allowing the content to fit in realistically with information and questions from the patient or virtual doctor. The frequent dialogue between the student, patient, and doctor provides a very high level of interactivity to make the cases both interesting and engaging.

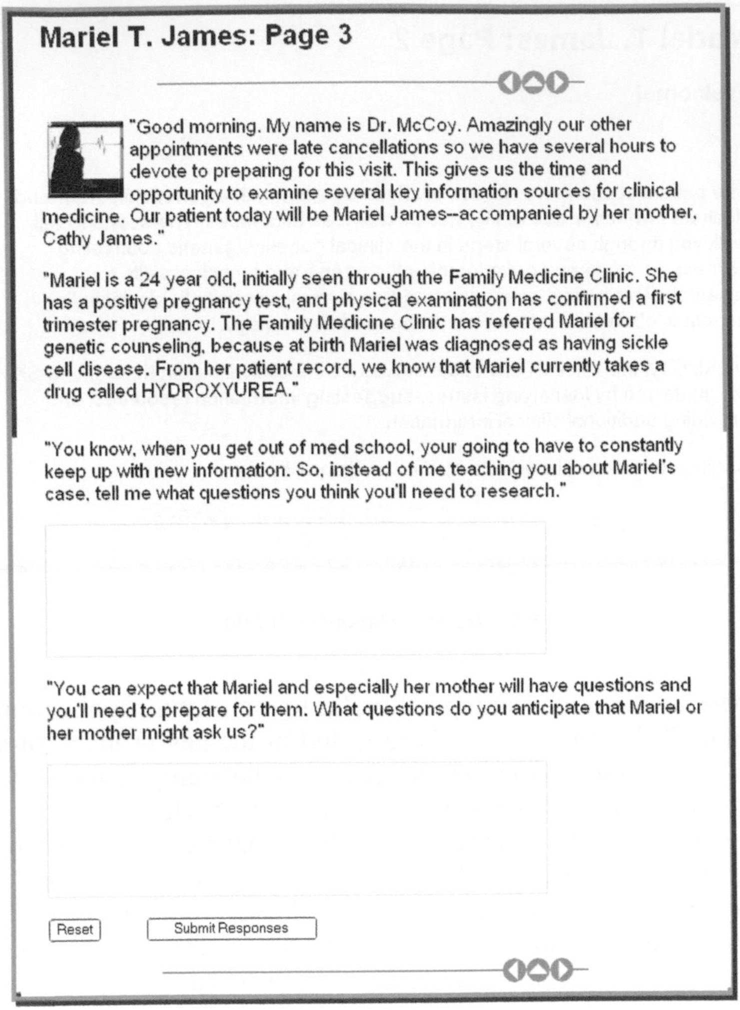

Mariel T. James: Page 3

---◀◐▶-

"Good morning. My name is Dr. McCoy. Amazingly our other appointments were late cancellations so we have several hours to devote to preparing for this visit. This gives us the time and opportunity to examine several key information sources for clinical medicine. Our patient today will be Mariel James--accompanied by her mother, Cathy James."

"Mariel is a 24 year old, initially seen through the Family Medicine Clinic. She has a positive pregnancy test, and physical examination has confirmed a first trimester pregnancy. The Family Medicine Clinic has referred Mariel for genetic counseling, because at birth Mariel was diagnosed as having sickle cell disease. From her patient record, we know that Mariel currently takes a drug called HYDROXYUREA."

"You know, when you get out of med school, your going to have to constantly keep up with new information. So, instead of me teaching you about Mariel's case, tell me what questions you think you'll need to research."

"You can expect that Mariel and especially her mother will have questions and you'll need to prepare for them. What questions do you anticipate that Mariel or her mother might ask us?"

[Reset]   [Submit Responses]

---◀◐▶-

FIGURE 9.3. Beginning of case details and dialogue.

Recall of Prior Learning

A brief multiple-choice quiz is included within the case study, to stimulate recall of what students already understand about MED-LINE and MeSH. A similar short quiz precedes each of the databases used in the course. Students evaluate their scores and are advised to

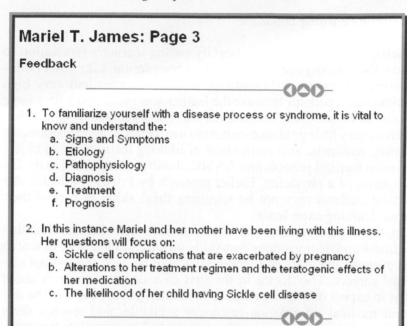

Mariel T. James: Page 3

Feedback

1. To familiarize yourself with a disease process or syndrome, it is vital to know and understand the:
   a. Signs and Symptoms
   b. Etiology
   c. Pathophysiology
   d. Diagnosis
   e. Treatment
   f. Prognosis

2. In this instance Mariel and her mother have been living with this illness. Her questions will focus on:
   a. Sickle cell complications that are exacerbated by pregnancy
   b. Alterations to her treatment regimen and the teratogenic effects of her medication
   c. The likelihood of her child having Sickle cell disease

FIGURE 9.4. Standardized feedback.

take the tutorial if they score poorly. As adult learners, students are expected to make the decision whether or not to complete the tutorials or continue with the case studies. They are advised that the short time spent with each tutorial will reduce their time obtaining and evaluating relevant search results.

Presenting the Content

A case study format allowed the authors to embed the knowledge and skill components into an investigative storytelling method. Educational research suggests that storytelling is a particularly effective method of learning and may even be "hardwired" into people as a part of human evolution.[6] Case studies may also provide an appropriate learning context for activities taking place later in a clinical setting.

Providing Learning Guidance

Self-paced learning relies heavily on the learner's motivation to follow the learning exercise through to completion. Like older correspondence courses, early distance learning courses had very high dropout rates, perhaps because the learner was presented with a large amount of instructional content that was not organized well, and they received very little guidance on how to use it effectively. Self-directed learning readiness, as a component of lifelong learning, is an objective most medical schools and AAMC identify as important in the development of a physician. Earlier research by Frisby[7] indicates that medical students may not be acquiring these skills as part of their formal learning experience.

In these case studies, the doctor models self-directed learning readiness and demonstrates that skills acquired in learning to search and evaluate the medical literature that will be used throughout students' careers. The doctor in the first case coaches students about what to expect during the clinical encounter, guides them to the different medical information resources available, and teaches them which resource is appropriate for each task. The virtual doctor models the learning behavior Jefferson wants its students to acquire. Later case studies remove this structured guidance, forcing students to reflect on what they did on the previous case, analyze what the problem calls for in the new case, and apply those skills to reach a solution. The repetition of this process provides additional reinforcement designed to increase students' self-confidence in their own readiness for self-directed learning. As shown in Figure 9.5, students are asked to apply their new skills in searching MEDLINE in general to a specific search for evidence-based articles using the limit command.

The case study continues (Figure 9.6) by asking the student to investigate any complications associated with the suggested treatment. This begins with an assessment of the student's current knowledge and skill using the MICROMEDEX database. After evaluating his or her performance, a student may choose to use the MICROMEDEX tutorial, and then continue with the case study.

Elicit Performance

Frequent interaction between the student and the doctor provides motivation and continued coaching throughout the case. Although

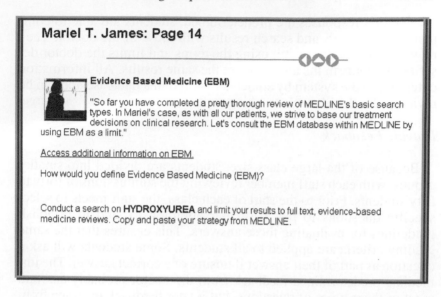

FIGURE 9.5. Limiting MEDLINE results to evidence-based medicine reviews.

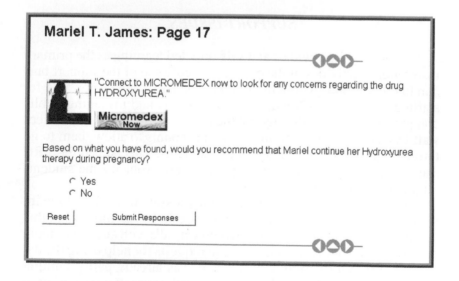

FIGURE 9.6. Making decisions based on information retrieved.

the doctor's responses are predetermined, students are able to compare their answers and search results with those of the doctor. They may also repeat the search using the terms and limits the doctor describes to confirm the ability to get the same results. All information entered into the system by students is stored in a database and can be reviewed by the library's teaching staff.

Provide Feedback

Because of the large class size, students are divided into smaller groups, with each staff member reviewing the submissions of forty to fifty students. Prior to the start of each class, the staff meets to select specific questions to pay particular attention to, and to establish guidelines for evaluating those answers. This ensures that the same grading criteria are applied to all students. Some students will ask a question as part of their answer if unsure of a correct answer. The immediate predetermined feedback from the doctor probably answers most of these types of questions, but a later feedback message from one of the library's teaching staff provides additional information and reinforcement.

SUPPORT ISSUES

The move to case studies and self-directed learning as the primary instructional activities of the course shifted some of the support burden to other groups within the library. The LRCs are responsible for staffing the university's computer classrooms and managing public computers distributed throughout the library. The Education Services staff trained the LRC staff and created accounts to allow them to go through the course in advance of the students. This helped the LRC staff to answer questions and respond to any problems the students might encounter in completing the exercises.

Other groups affected were the library's systems staff and the information services staff at the reference desk. It was anticipated that the reference desk, like the LRC, would get calls with questions about the cases and would see an increase in requests for help using the databases. The information services staff was already partly familiar with the course, as they assisted in writing the pool of questions used in the pre- and post-tests. Course accounts were also created for members of the information services staff, giving them the opportunity to complete the case studies and become familiar with the exercises.

With permission from the database vendors, the systems staff mapped the students' individual accounts for database access to a special training account during the course period. This protects Jefferson's hospital and research users from being denied access to resources with a limited number of simultaneous users.

Instructional Event

Assess Performance

In addition to completing the two required case studies in the course, students take a post-test exam. The average post-test score was 90, an improvement of 21 points above the pre-test average of 68 (both out of a possible 100 points for twenty questions). Students are skeptical about the pre-test at the start of the course, since they are not commonly used in their other courses. Exemplifying the competitiveness of medical school, students occasionally request to retake the pre-test because they think they did poorly.

Enhance Retention and Transfer

The first case study ends with a short summary of the purpose of the case study in relation to the course objectives. The next case study adds two additional databases to the scenario, allowing the student to practice what has been learned so far and apply it to similar situations. During the course, the teaching team frequently checks the database for student answers to questions and scans for anomalies or questions within the answers. Feedback is given as appropriate. One week following the course, a final message is sent to the class regarding their overall performance and addressing two or three areas that have similar patterns of misunderstanding. In one example from a previous year regarding diabetes and scuba diving, many students submitted an incorrect answer based on information from a site found by using a general Internet search engine, which listed that site near the top of the list. This indicates a continuing problem with reliance on general Internet search engines instead of appropriate clinical resources.

EVALUATION METHODS

This course provides frequent self-assessment. Students complete a pre-test to objectively measure baseline knowledge about using databases to locate medical information. As part of the case studies, students encounter several small quizzes that evaluate their understanding of how to structure search questions, choose a database appropriate for the question, and execute a search in that database. Students score these quizzes for themselves and determine whether or not they should complete the associated tutorials. As with all self-directed learning, this puts the responsibility for learning on the student—where it will be when he or she is a practicing physician. The last formal assessment is the post-test. Again, students were presented with a set of questions from the same pool used in the pre-test. The course management program allows for the items to be presented randomly (both question order and choice options), and the final score is immediately available to each student.

The last requirement is the completion of the course evaluation. This allows students to comment on the effectiveness of the orientation session, on the use of case studies as a vehicle for learning medical informatics, and on levels of satisfaction in the course as a whole. Scores for these measures range from 80 to 90 percent (good to excellent). Results from the 2003 course determined that only 25 percent of the students rated their current searching skills as good or excellent before the course compared to 87 percent on the postcourse evaluation. In addition, 99 percent of the postcourse respondents considered these skills highly relevant to their career as a physician and 98 percent considered them relevant to their success as medical students.

Results indicate that this course format is effective and appropriate for teaching information literacy skills to medical students. The team hopes that the knowledge and skills acquired by the students during the course are retained and available for use when needed later in clinical practice. This retention is something Jefferson is just beginning to assess in its graduates.

FUTURE PLANS

The students' high level of satisfaction with this course has helped to promote the development of similar materials for additional courses in both Jefferson Medical College and the Jefferson College of Health Professions. The Education Services team is currently exploring the idea of building an OSCE (Objective Structured Clinical Exam) case study for the medical college that will require students to consult the literature for evidence-based medicine solutions.

Researchers at Jefferson Medical College's Center for Research in Medical Education and Health Care and Dr. Frisby have been working on an instrument to measure lifelong learning attitudes and skills in Jefferson graduates. A survey instrument was developed in 2002 and tested on several smaller populations.[8] It is hoped that survey results for graduates will indicate an upward trend in attitude and skills for self-directed lifelong learning.

Developing realistic, interactive case studies is time-consuming and requires a team approach. Team members averaged 200 hours of work per one hour of finished online activity. Pairing professional librarians, educators, and experts in the target field is necessary to construct cases that are convincing to students. In Jefferson's experience, the results are worth the effort.

NOTES

1. Gagne, R.M., Briggs, L.J., and Wagner, W.W. *Principles of Instructional Design.* New York: Holt, Rinehart and Winston, 1988.

2. Gagne, R.M. *The Conditions of Learning and Theory of Instruction.* New York: Holt, Rinehart and Winston, 1985.

3. Association of American Medical Colleges. *Learning Objectives for Medical Student Education: Guidelines for Medical Schools.* Washington, DC: Association of American Medical Colleges, 1998. Available: <http://www.aamc.org/meded/msop/msop1.pdf>.

4. American Association of School Librarians and Association for Educational Communications and Technology. *American Library Association Information Literacy Standards for Student Learning.* Chicago: American Library Association, 1998. Available: <http://www.ala.org/aasl/ip_nine. html>.

5. Brown, J.S., Collins, A., and Duguid, S. "Situated Cognition and the Culture of Learning." *Educational Researcher* 18(1988):32-42.

6. Brown, J.S. and Duguid, P. *The Social Life of Information.* Boston, MA: Harvard Business School Press, 2000.

7. Frisby, A.J. "Self-Directed Learning Readiness in Medical Students at The Ohio State University." Ann Arbor, MI: Dissertation Abstracts International, 1991.

8. Hojat, M., Nasca, T.J., Erdmann, J.B., Frisby, A.J., Veloski, J.J., and Connella, J.S. "An Operational Measure of Physician Lifelong Learning: Its Development, Components and Preliminary Psychometric Data." *Medical Teacher* 26(July 2003): 433-437.

Chapter 10

Education and E-Learning at the William H. Welch Medical Library

Cynthia L. Sheffield
Jayne M. Campbell
Dongming Zhang

INTRODUCTION

The William H. Welch Medical Library offers a variety of educational opportunities for faculty, staff, and students affiliated with the Johns Hopkins Medical Institutions. Welch Medical Library staff use the scientific communication process as the framework for identifying content. Teaching formats vary depending on expressed user needs, audience, and available technologies. Classroom-based course content <http://www.welch.jhu.edu/classes/> is offered through three distinct yet interrelated programs: *Resources for Research, Information Management and Presentation; e-Welch: Introduction and Update on the Library;* and *Computer and Communication Technologies.* Most recently, the focus has been on the development of the e-learning Web site <http://www.welch.jhu.edu/classes/elearning/>. As shown in Figure 10.1, content is delivered using online tutorials, handouts, links to lectures and classes, and more. This chapter describes the genesis of these education programs and development of content within the context of the underlying technologies and databases.

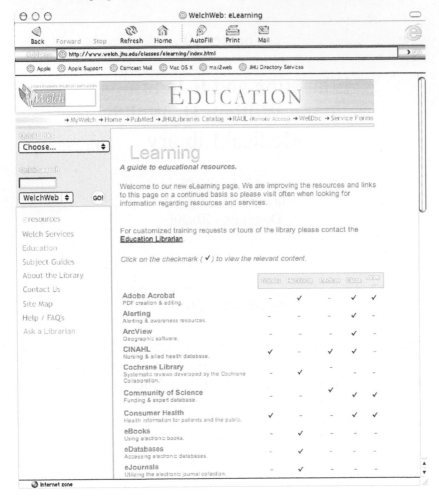

FIGURE 10.1. E-learning index page.

SETTING

The Johns Hopkins University, founded by a Quaker merchant in Baltimore, has a long history as a leader in teaching and research. The Division of Health Sciences Informatics is an academic unit that encompasses the library, informatics research, and informatics education. Goals include the development and use of electronic and other information resources for decision making, research, health care delivery, and individual academic growth, and increasing the awareness of these resources throughout the medical institutions.

Welch Medical Library, the central component of the division, provides information services and educational programs that advance research, teaching, and patient care. WelchWeb <http://www.welch.jhu.edu/>, the library's Web site, serves as the front door to the complete array of library programs and services (see Figure 10.2). The Welch Medical Library subscribes to approximately 2,700 electronic

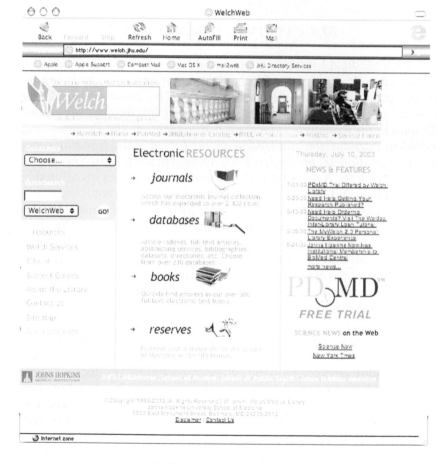

FIGURE 10.2. WelchWeb.

journals and maintains a modest print collection as it transitions into a world in which the entire collection will be available electronically.

The Welch Medical Library's potential user group consists of over 30,000 individuals affiliated with the Johns Hopkins Medical Institutions, in various locations throughout the Baltimore metropolitan region. Affiliated institutions include the Johns Hopkins Hospital, Bayview Medical Center, Howard County Community Hospital, Kennedy Krieger Institute, and all of their affiliated outpatient centers, as well as the Johns Hopkins University School of Medicine, School of Nursing, and the Bloomberg School of Public Health.

EDUCATIONAL APPROACHES

Welch Medical Library's educational program is designed around tools and technologies for biomedical communication and support of the scientific communication process. Classroom-based course content is offered through three distinct yet interrelated programs: *Resources for Research, Information Management and Presentation*; *e-Welch: Introduction and Update on the Library*; and *Computer and Communication Technologies*. Participation in the first two programs is free of charge. A registration fee is applied to the courses offered in the computer and communication technologies program.

The courses offered in *Resources for Research, Information Management and Presentation* are the cornerstone of the entire education program. Content is selected from a broad range of topics, including database searching, managing scientific references, writing a grant application or research paper, finding funding, keeping up-to-date with the research literature, and understanding the basic concepts and resources for evidence-based health care.

e-Welch: Introduction and Update on the Library is a regular lecture series concerning topics important to its user community (see Figure 10.3). These lectures are offered to all Hopkins affiliates and do not require advance registration. Lecture content is selected to provide an introduction to topics that are more broadly presented in other teaching forums. Lectures offer faculty, staff, and students an opportunity to learn about new and existing services and technologies provided by the library. Topics include research resources, database searching, managing scientific references, evidence-based health care, complementary and alternative medicine, and pharmacology resources.

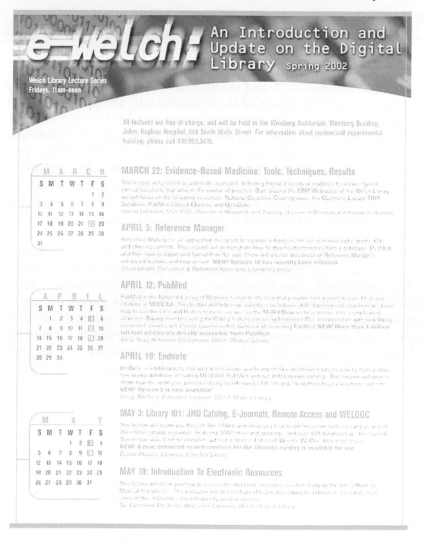

FIGURE 10.3. e-Welch library lecture series.

The *Computer and Communication Technologies* program covers productivity applications such as database programs, spreadsheets, presentation and slide making, word processing, and the Adobe Acrobat PDF work environment.

E-Learning

Developing an e-learning site was a natural progression from the established course offerings and lecture series. Hopkins physicians, nurses, technicians, staff, and students work varying shifts, often far from the library. For many of these individuals, attending hands-on classes or lectures is difficult, if not impossible.

Detailed class booklets support most of the hands-on classes and are often used as stand-alone instruction manuals. PowerPoint presentations also support the content of each topic within the lecture series, which can be enough information to get users started on their research or give an overview of a particular database. In addition to the booklets and slides developed in-house, links are created to online tutorials and instruction guides created by database suppliers.

The ability to get instruction anytime, anywhere makes e-learning appealing to many information users. Electronic instruction or distance education is a much more acceptable format for learning. Windows 95 revolutionized distance education. Before its release, enormous amounts of development time were necessary to produce tutorials that would work; at best, most tutorials only worked in a finite set of operating systems. To make matters worse, system requirements and standards fluctuated, making the viability of any well-developed tutorial questionable. In addition, users needed a modest level of computer experience to navigate programs successfully, although the tutorials were intended to help novices. Once Windows set the standard, new software became available, making the design and development of learning modules much easier. Audio and video components can be produced at a fraction of the former cost, both in terms of labor invested and the cost of the software itself. With the use of readily available plug-ins, e-learning modules appeal to visual, auditory, and tactile learners alike.

At the library, each instructor is responsible for his or her content area of the Web site in terms of design, development, and updates. Several staff training sessions established a baseline of familiarity with technical applications and processes used. These sessions were also used to establish goals and expectations for developers. Content experts often work in teams to support specific topics, resulting in better input for the design, a natural peer review process, and additional staff to answer questions about each learning module. Adequate coverage is necessary to resolve any problems e-learners may have regarding systems.

Users may already feel slightly removed by virtue of remote access. In a reference area or classroom setting, experienced instructors can sense when a student is having trouble. In a remote environment, users ask questions and expect a timely answer. Remote users can become frustrated and move on to something else, possibly losing the teachable moment.

Another benefit to having a team of instructors providing support is that it allows professionals and paraprofessionals alike to increase their skills in that content area. Each time a process is reviewed, a system's capability is tested, or a technical problem is resolved, this experience expands staff knowledge of that particular subject. Staff members can also increase their knowledge base by assisting in the training lab or with the lecture series. These opportunities allow staff members to review the content, become comfortable with the instructional environment, and see a wide variety of trouble spots and questions relevant to that software or database. Ultimately this information can be used to improve existing instruction modules.

Designing the presentation of information about e-learning was one of the most critical and difficult steps in the development process. Welch Medical Library users vary from the most experienced academics to novice users returning to research after several years away from formalized education. Experienced researchers tend to have very specific questions but may need to become familiar with recent changes in a specific database such as PubMed. Inexperienced users may require detailed instructions on several Welch systems and how these systems relate to each other. It is easy to adjust to learner knowledge when interacting in person, but it is more difficult to develop an asynchronous instruction stance that reaches everyone. Instructions written for adept users can confuse new learners, and instructions written for new users can frustrate more experienced users. In an effort to reach both types of learners, it was decided to list subjects alphabetically for the first rendition of e-learning. Titles for subject areas were carefully selected to reflect the most popular terminology based on content. In many cases, overlap occurs among subject areas.

The overall appearance of the site was addressed during the design phase. It was important for each content area to have a sense of cohesion, helping users associate each module as belonging to the e-learning page, and to facilitate easy navigation among the modules. To accomplish this, the Welch Medical Library's graphic artist designed a template, which created standardization for the format and development of modules (see Figure 10.4). Standardization makes it easier for each designer to plan the content and address specific areas of the learning process. For instance, each module has a place for an introduction, follow-up contact information, learning exercises, and options for the learner to practice new skills. Instructors can create as many module sections as needed to describe content.

E-Learning Development Tools

The technologies for Internet and Web development have grown at a rapid pace during the past decade and are used for creating, developing, and delivering Internet e-learning content and modules. Standardized technologies ensure that tools, delivery methods, and formats

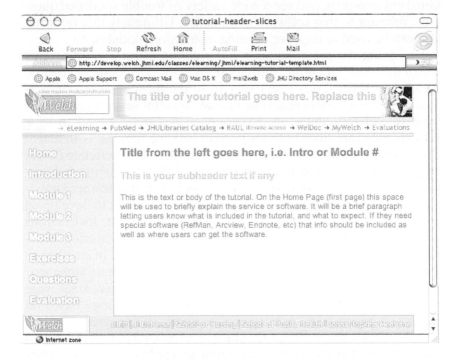

FIGURE 10.4. E-learning template.

can be integrated as new technologies are developed and established. These technologies are involved in creating generic text, generic image/graphic, user interfaces, and the e-learning services environment.

The most commonly used software for generic text creation includes Word, Adobe Acrobat, and PowerPoint. These tools create files that can be deployed on generic Web servers or file servers that Web/application servers access and fetch. Users can download these files through Internet access or open files directly using browser-embedded plug-in software.

Generic image/graphic creation software includes Photoshop, Fireworks, and others. Content developed by these graphic tools can be embedded or integrated with the generic text files described previously or can be independently deployed on Web servers, downloadable by users.

Multimedia creation software include Flash, Director, Streaming Video, and Real software. These highly graphic images use audio, video, and animation as their presentation formats. Similar to other Internet files, these files can be deployed on Web servers and are viewable via browser-embedded plug-in software. The skills required for using the software are relatively greater than the skills necessary for other software.

Simulation creation usually refers to the creation of two-dimensional or three-dimensional virtual reality in which the learning contents are presented in an intuitive, lifelike fashion. Current commonly used software includes regular professional programming languages such as Java, C++, C, and Visual Basic. Sometimes the creation process involves other multimedia and image software, such as Flash and Photoshop. This is the most complex process for creating learning contents and usually requires a team comprising content developers, software engineers, and graphic/multimedia designers. Simulation learning content can be deployed on the Web servers or delivered using CD/DVD as the media.

The design and development of Web interfaces is an important factor in the success of e-learning services. Appealing user interfaces will immediately attract the attention of users and sustain their interest in further exploring the site. Interface design includes clean layouts, reasonable content organization, graphic-assisted directions, and efficient search engines. Usability testing and evaluation are necessary to ensure user satisfaction. The tools used to develop interfaces are varied and include the image/graphic tools just discussed. The most commonly used search engines include Inktomi, Ultraseek, Google, and specific SQL database engines (Oracle, SQL, Access).

The best Web environment for e-learning services is one in which the individual user can access learning material, complete online evaluations and quizzes, and download or save information for later review. Database and Web/application technology are crucial for storing user credentials for authentication, course information and content, evaluation and quiz data, and business rules that manage and maintain the whole site. An application server plays a middle-tier function that analyzes user input, interacts with the database, and delivers results to the user. The most commonly used databases are Oracle, SQL, and Access and the most commonly used application development tools are ColdFusion, ASP, JSP, and programming languages such as Perl, C, C++, and Java.

E-learning file format standards relate to the correct download and use by local software. Since most local desktops are Windows-based or Macintosh OS X-based, formats of downloaded files need to be compatible with the capability of the local desktop. Regular files include Word, PowerPoint, Adobe Acrobat PDF, and JPEG/MPEG/GIF. PostScript and TIFF formatted files may need extra conversion or other software to be accessed.

Users should be able to interact with course contents on the system that best meets their immediate needs. An e-learning system can determine a course package based on course contents and the requests, backgrounds, aptitudes, and previous learning profiles of users. It should provide an appropriate user evaluation mechanism to assist in regular improvement of course contents. User profiles, including professional interests, can help identify contents and services needed to improve the quality of the service.

E-Learning User Interfaces

A well-designed interface is an important factor in the success of e-learning services. An appealing user interface will attract and sustain the attention of users. Interface design includes clean layouts, reasonable content organization, graphic-assisted directions, and efficient search engines that allow users to quickly locate what is needed. Usability testing and evaluation are necessary to ensure users' satisfaction.

FUTURE PLANS

The development of the e-learning site is a work in progress. Goals for the future include:

- developing a content management system to manage global updates;
- developing a systematic peer review process to ensure quality control;
- providing a mechanism to collect user feedback about the learning experience;
- formalizing commitments from content developers so that expectations are understood and met;
- developing search engines and lexicons to locate specific attributes within content areas;
- tracking selected links and site searches, feedback, questions submitted, and answers to practice exercises; and
- further developing the technical skills of library staff to enhance the level of service provided by the Web site.

CONCLUSION

Welch Medical Library's existing education program provides a broad range of library-related classes, a lecture series to highlight these information topics, and productivity applications. This foundation is being used to broaden user groups by making instructional materials available to anyone, anytime, anywhere. Library staff members have developed materials that can be applied to a distance education or e-learning environment. Technical factors concerning the content, user interface, service environment, and delivery all need to be made with careful deliberation, as they will affect not only current site development but future development as well. This e-learning site is an efficient tool for keeping a large user community current with changes to health sciences information and resources. Goals for the future of this site continue to evolve as current stages of this project unfold.

Chapter 11

An Informatics Course
for First-Year Pharmacy Students
at the University of California,
San Francisco

David J. Owen
Gail L. Persily
Patricia C. Babbitt

INTRODUCTION

The current technological revolution is rapidly changing the face of health care delivery, with the Internet profoundly affecting the practice and business of pharmacy.[1] Advances in information technology are likely to continue unabated, so that today's pharmacists will encounter computerized resources and tools throughout their educational and professional careers. As pharmacy moves into the twenty-first century, and as the health care scene evolves in response to these and other changes, it is imperative that pharmacists learn how to make effective use of the new resources and understand how information technology is being used to facilitate patient care.

The increasing ubiquity of computerized systems in health care has led to the emergence of a new specialty, termed "medical informatics" or "health care informatics." As defined by the Association of American Medical Colleges, medical informatics is

> a developing body of knowledge and a set of techniques concerning the organizational management of information in support of medical research, education, and patient care. . . . Medical informatics combines medical science with several

technologies and disciplines in the information and computer sciences and provides methodologies by which these can contribute to better use of the medical knowledge base and ultimately to better medical care.[2]

Similarly, pharmacy informatics aims at training the pharmacist to understand how to use the new information tools to aid in the delivery of pharmaceutical knowledge for optimal patient care. Not only does it cover drug information sources and systematic drug literature searches, but it also requires a basic understanding of clinical information systems, Web page construction and design, multimedia applications, database constructions, use of biomedical and genomic sequencing databases, government regulation of medical information, health literacy, and evaluation studies, as well as exposure to different pharmacy systems currently available.[3]

Libraries are similarly redefining their traditional roles in response to developments in information technology and are taking on a more dynamic role in the new information-intensive environment.[4] As information professionals, librarians have expertise in information classification, information retrieval, and the construction and use of controlled vocabularies. Most libraries are now actively involved in the development and teaching of information literacy courses. The National Library of Medicine is a leader in such educational efforts, providing financial support for research and teaching in medical informatics, and sponsoring a variety of training programs for health professionals and individuals working in the biomedical sciences. This chapter discusses the contribution of librarians to the design and implementation of an innovative pharmacy informatics course at the University of California, San Francisco (UCSF).

SETTING

UCSF is one of ten campuses in the University of California (UC) public university system, and is the only UC campus devoted solely to the health sciences. UCSF includes professional schools of dentistry, medicine, nursing, and pharmacy; a graduate division for predoctoral and postdoctoral scientists; UCSF Medical Center; UCSF Children's Hospital; and Langley Porter Psychiatric Institute. The UCSF Kalmanovitz Library serves 3,500 students and supports the teaching, research, and service missions of the campus. The library's Education Services unit consists of three education coordinators with liaison responsibilities to the academic schools and programs.

In 1998, the UCSF School of Pharmacy launched a new curriculum, designed to provide a program that better prepares PharmD graduates for the changing health care environment. The new curriculum emphasizes the role of pharmacists as information providers, the importance of a commitment to lifelong learning, and includes among its stated goals the use of informatics and information management in pharmacy practice and research. As part of its commitment to curriculum-integrated instruction, the UCSF library was invited to contribute course sections on information resources, focusing not only on online information resources for pharmacy and pharmaceuticals but also on the fundamentals of database management systems.

EDUCATIONAL APPROACHES

As part of its new curriculum, the School of Pharmacy wanted to include a required first-year course focusing on informatics topics of relevance to pharmacists. Initially, pharmacy students attended a course offered through the School of Nursing, but evaluations showed that students found the material too theoretical and they seemed unable to understand its application to pharmacy. In spring 1999, Dr. Patricia Babbitt, associate professor in the Departments of Biopharmaceutical Sciences and Pharmaceutical Chemistry, and the newly appointed course director, called a meeting of interested parties to discuss the creation of a new course specifically for the PharmD program. Dr. Babbitt assembled a multidisciplinary group of pharmacy faculty, librarians, researchers, clinical information specialists, basic science researchers, and clinical pharmacy practitioners to brainstorm about the new course. The meeting focused on designing a syllabus that would present material in an engaging and coherent manner and would illustrate how the clinical pharmacist uses informatics in practice.

The group set the following course goal: "training tomorrow's pharmacists in the fundamentals of practicing pharmacy in the informatics age." To achieve these goals, Dr. Babbitt created a ten-week, three-unit course, *Introduction to Pharmacy Informatics* (hereafter referred to by its course number, BPS114). Topics covered in lecture and lab sessions include online pharmacy and pharmaceutical information resources for pharmacists; introduction to structured vocabularies and their importance in accessing drug information; evidence-based health care and the Cochrane Library; using a hospital pharmacy database; consumer drug information; and drug resources and tools for personal digital assistants (PDAs) and other handheld devices. Specific lecture/lab sessions include the following:

- Online Library Resources
- Structured Vocabularies
- Database Principles and Design
- Computer-Based Patient Record System (CPR), Electronic Medical Records (EMR), or Electronic Patient Records (EPR)
- Clinical Pharmacy Databases
- Integrated Health Information Systems
- Privacy, Security and Confidentiality
- The Cochrane Collaboration
- Introduction to MICROMEDEX
- Providing Drug Information over the Internet
- The California Poison Control System
- Developing an Online Drug Information Page
- Telepharmacy
- PDAs for Pharmacists
- Automation in Pharmacy
- Computational Drug Design
- The Human Genome Project
- Pharmacogenomics

In addition to faculty in the School of Pharmacy, guest speakers were identified to discuss specific implementations of systems relevant to pharmacy.

The course consists of two lecture hours per week and a three-hour hands-on computer lab to complement the lecture content. This lecture/lab combination was devised as the key strategy to help students understand the practical application of the lecture topics to pharmacy practice. Faculty, librarians, researchers, and practitioners with expertise in the topic areas provide the lectures. The course director also lectures and attends every session to introduce the lectures and provide the context and unifying themes for the course. The hands-on computer lab sessions that accompany most of the lectures provide a central element of the course. In the laboratory, students gain experience using information technology and database systems, including retrieving information from online bibliographic databases and key drug information resources; creation of a simple database and data manipulation; design and construction of Web pages to simulate responses to patient queries; and use and applications of a clinical pharmacy database.

BPS114 uses WebCT, an online course management system, to deliver course information, lecture notes, assignments, and other information supplemental to in-class instruction. At UCSF, WebCT is used by all professional schools and the graduate division to support graduate medical education. The library manages WebCT for the campus through its Center for Instructional Technology (CIT). The CIT is part of the library's education services and therefore provides additional opportunities to collaborate with faculty on their courses.

BPS114 was first offered in spring quarter 2000 and is now a requirement for all first-year pharmacy students. The lab sessions, offered in six sections to accommodate all 120 students, are held in the Thomas A. Oliver Informatics Resource Center, a state-of-the-art computer lab in the School of Pharmacy. A graduate teaching assistant usually helps the instructors with each lab session. The course structure and content have remained essentially the same since the course's inception, although there have been slight modifications each year in response to new technological developments or changes in subject emphasis that reflect the primary interests of different invited lecturers. This case study describes the library's role in the course as offered from 2001 to 2003.

The Library's Role

The course director contacted UCSF librarians for contributions to BPS114 as a result of previous successful collaborations between the library and School of Pharmacy related to basic database design and information organization and retrieval. The library collaborated on three components of BPS114: (1) searching for drug information using controlled vocabularies, (2) database principles and design, and

(3) applying a conceptual model for drug information to clinical pharmacy.

The first computer lab session was devoted mostly to the importance of the primary literature and effective search strategies for retrieving information from the MEDLINE database on the PubMed system. A key concept of the informatics course is the importance of controlled vocabularies such as Medical Subject Headings (MeSH) in locating drug information. Controlled or structured vocabularies are covered in the second lecture and are emphasized throughout the course. In addition to MEDLINE, their use is illustrated in various applications and databases including the indexing of the published biomedical literature and drug information systems.

Although concentrating on the effective use of MeSH for drug information retrieval, the first lab taught by librarians introduces students to a core group of bibliographic databases and important online drug reference tools as a way to not only show the variety of resources available for pharmacy information but to demonstrate some of the different controlled vocabularies employed by bibliographic databases. The following resources—all available through GALEN II, the digital library of UCSF—were demonstrated: BIOSIS Previews, Current Contents, Science Citation Index, Drug Information Full-Text (DIF), Cochrane Library, and International Pharmaceutical Abstracts (IPA). Students are first taught the basics of searching MEDLINE, with an emphasis on understanding the use of MeSH and subheadings to retrieve drug information. Sample exercise questions include:

- *What is the MeSH term for over-the-counter drugs?* (Designed to show the concept of a controlled vocabulary and how this is related to mapping by the PubMed search engine)
- *The MeSH term "Drugs, Non-Prescription" is part of which broader category?* (Designed to show the MeSH tree structures)
- *Display all MeSH terms in the broader category for "Drugs, Non-Prescription." How does the scope note define "Investigational Drugs"?* (Designed to get students to navigate and explore related branches of the MeSH tree)

The IPA Database, produced by the American Society of Health-Systems Pharmacists (ASHSP), also uses a controlled vocabulary with a combination of broad and specific index terms. Although the thesaurus is not as sophisticated or as comprehensive as MeSH, the narrower subject scope of the IPA thesaurus allows use of pharmacy-specific terminology and a greater degree of specificity at which concepts are defined. To demonstrate this, students are asked to run the same searches in both PubMed and IPA, and then compare and contrast subject headings affixed to records retrieved for the topic "consumer use of the Internet to purchase prescription drugs." Table 11.1 illustrates the results of this exercise.

The IPA database and the full-text resource DIF are both produced by the ASHSP and both employ the American Hospital Formulary System (AHFS) Pharmacologic-Therapeutic Classification scheme to aid in information retrieval. Students were asked to examine the Therapeutic Classification field in both databases. This drug classification system is an important example of a different classification scheme widely used in pharmacies to classify drug information systems such as hospital formularies. Exercises were designed to show the unique characteristics and strengths of using the AHFS classification terms in each resource.

TABLE 11.1. Comparing and contrasting MEDLINE/IPA indexing terms.

Database	Thesaurus	Indexing terms
MEDLINE	MeSH	(1) Pharmaceutical preparations (2) Internet (3) Drugs, Prescription
IPA	IPA thesaurus	(1) Prescription Drugs (2) Internet (Prescription Drugs) (3) Prescribing (Internet) (4) Pharmacy (Practice) (5) Crime (Prescription Drugs) (6) Computers (Internet) (7) Internet (Dispensing) (8) Regulations (Internet) (9) Sales (Prescription Drugs) (10) World Wide Web (Prescription Drugs) (11) Pharmacy, Community (Internet)

Note: Indexing terms attached to records retrieved for the search "consumer use of the Internet to purchase prescription drugs."

As previously mentioned, information retrieval from PubMed using the MeSH vocabulary served as a useful introduction to the concept of controlled or structured vocabularies in the biomedical sciences. Drug vocabulary development and management is an important topic in pharmacy informatics that has far-reaching implications for the practice of medicine in general and drug therapy in particular. Discussing this topic early in the course, during the PubMed lab sessions, served as a useful introduction to the more advanced topic of concept-based controlled drug vocabularies in computerized drug information systems. This topic is covered in greater detail in a lecture and associated computer labs centered on the First DataBank drug information system.

For the second section of the course, *Database Principles and Design,* librarians designed and presented both lecture and computer lab. This part of the course was designed to provide pharmacy students with a basic understanding of databases and database design. The lecture emphasized defining a database, how it works, and how different users interact with databases. If students understand the structure behind databases, they can use information systems more effectively, work more effectively with systems developers and vendors, and design their own databases. Because of the ubiquity and importance of the relational database model, the lecture and lab focused on its key features of normalization, related tables, and the use of the structured query language to retrieve information. The computer lab session provided students with hands-on experience creating a table, linking up tables, and retrieving information from the database through the creation of the Access Simple Query function. Simple three-table relational databases were constructed for the lab exercises. As shown in Figure 11.1, a hypothetical pharmacy inventory centered on dietary supplements such as herbs and vitamins, a topic known to be of great interest to pharmacy students.

Using Simple Query, students are asked to construct simple searches to answer a list of questions (Figure 11.2) such as: *Which customers bought vitamins? Who manufactures the creatine supplement? Which is the most expensive herbal product?*

Students found the hands-on Access lab engaging and useful. These Access labs serve not only as an introduction to relational databases but prepare them for a more advanced lab held the following week, which requires creation of more advanced queries in associa-

Table 1: Customer Information

	CustomerID	FirstName	LastName	Street	City	Product
▶	1	Susan	Lee	High Street	Oakland	Breathe Easy
	2	Alan	Smith	Willow Avenue	Oakland	Senile Delight
	3	Min-Lin	Fang	9th Avenue	San Francisco	Breathe Easy
	4	Morgan	Fairchild	4th Street	San Francisco	Actival
	5	Manual	Gonsalez	Valencia Avenu	San Francisco	Young Again
	6	Helen	Ready	High Street	Oakland	Lots of Hair

Table 2: Product Information

	ProductID	Product	Constituent	Form	Category	Price	Supplier
	1	Maxi-Muscle	Creatine	Capsule	Amino acid	$15.00	Nutrigen
	2	Breathe Easy	Echinacea	Tablet	Herb	$4.00	Natures Way
	3	ColdAway	Vitamin C	Solution	Vitamin	$5.00	AltMedCom
	4	NoWheeze	Ephedra	Tablet	Herb	$10.00	Natures Way
	5	SleepWell	Valerian	Powder	Herb	$6.00	Herberts Herbs
	6	Lots of Hair	Vitamin E	Capsule	Vitamin	$15.00	Nutrigen

Table 3: Supplier Information

	ID	Supplier	City	State	EMail
▶	1	Nutrigen	Petaluma	California	nutri@aol.com
	2	Natures Way	Fremont	California	nature@aol.com
	3	AltMedCom	Oakland	California	altmed@earthlink.com
	4	Herberts Herbs	Petaluma	California	herbie@maslink.com
	5	Carol's Creams	Sioux City	Iowa	carol@aol.com
	6	Veronica's Vitar	Los Angeles	California	wit@lanet.com

FIGURE 11.1. Access hypothetical relational database.

Simple Query to answer the question:
"Which customers use the product Boils-Be-Gone, and what is the price."

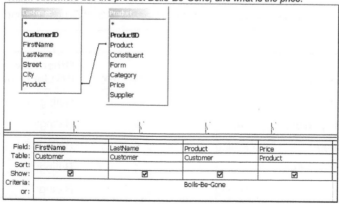

FIGURE 11.2. Creation of a Simple Query in Access.

tion with a clinical pharmacy information system developed by a UCSF pharmacist for use in her practice.

In the clinical pharmacy information system lab, students query a subset of a real clinical database, also using Access. They are able to focus on the content and structure of the information rather than the mechanics of the software.

In addition to the group computer lab sessions, some do-it-yourself labs were developed to provide some flexibility in the schedule. The library worked with the course director to develop one such lab to explore the application of controlled vocabularies to clinical pharmacy. Students are asked to read an article titled "A Concept-Based Medication Vocabulary: An Essential Requirement for Pharmacy Decision Support."[5] The article defines a concept-based model for describing drug information, which is based on the different information levels of any given drug. The levels include the basic ingredient set, clinical drug form and dosage, manufactured drug, and packaged drug. Building on prior lab sessions that covered MEDLINE, MICROMEDEX, and other resources, students ran searches on three drugs—an over-the-counter medication, an herbal supplement, and a prescription drug. Consult Table 11.2 and Box 11.1 for more information. The objective of the exercise was to rate various information sources according to concept levels of drugs defined by Broverman, and to illustrate the relative appropriateness of each source for locating the various types of information.

TABLE 11.2. Sample answer sheet for *Concept Levels of Drugs* assignment for diazepam.

Conceptual level	IPA	MICROMEDEX	Other resource (RxList or other)
Ingredient	Rating: 3	Rating: 5	Rating: 2
Generic ingredient set	Rating: 2	Rating: 4	Rating: 1
Clinical drug	Rating: 3	Rating: 5	Rating: 3
Manufactured drug	Rating: 2	Rating: 4	Rating: 3
Packaged drug product	Rating: 4	Rating: 3	Rating: 2

Rating: 1 = "Not very useful"; 5 = "Very useful"

BOX 11.1. Tips for Do-It-Yourself Resources

Read the Broverman et al. paper carefully before you begin the lab, so that you understand what the authors mean by referring to the five "Conceptual Levels of a Drug." Refer to the relevant sections and examples in the paper while completing the assignment.

Below is an example of a breakdown of the five conceptual levels for the drug Zantac. Notice that when we get to the clinical drug level, we specify the Zantac 150 Tablet. The remaining information is unique to that specific clinical drug.

ZANTAC

Ingredient	Ranitidine hydrochloride
Generic ingredient set	Ranitidine hydrochloride
Clinical drug	Available as tablets, capsules, as a syrup for people who have problems swallowing, or for intravenous injection. Specific clinical drug example would be Zantac 150 Tablet which contains 168 mg of ranitidine HCl equivalent to 150 mg of ranitidine
Manufactured drug	Glaxo Zantac 150 tablets are peach, film-coated, five-sided tablets embossed with "ZANTAC 150" on one side and "Glaxo" on the other. Inactive ingredients include aluminum lake, hydroxypropyl methylcellulose, magnesium stearate, microcrystalline cellulose, titanium dioxide, triacetin, and yellow iron oxide.
Packaged drug	Glaxo Zantac 150 Tablets are available in bottles of 30 (NDC 0173-0393-40) and 250 (NDC 0173-0393-06) tablets and unit dose packs of 100 (NDC 0173-0393-47) tablets.

Searching IPA

- Remember that there are a limited number of concurrent UCSF users, so you may not always be able to access the database.
- IPA uses a controlled vocabulary of terms that are found in the descriptor (DE) field. Display in the LONG format to view the DE field.
- There is no online thesaurus to browse, as in MEDLINE.
- Preference is for the generic drug name that can be found in the descriptor (DE) field.
- Drug trade names are included and can be found in the drug names (DR) field.

EVALUATION METHODS

Anecdotal student feedback allowed course developers to continually modify and improve the course each year. In general, feedback has been positive, and the comments received offer some insights and perspectives into the course's value to students. Typical comments include the following:

- "The structure of the class with a lecture and lab is a great idea."
- "I found some of the lectures difficult but I think I learned a lot about working with computers."
- "I was surprised how interesting this course was. It will really help me."
- "There was an interesting range of topics."
- "Most of the labs were interesting and I now know more about how computers will help me as a pharmacist."

Students commented on the usefulness of the Access sessions in preparing them for the more advanced labs and appreciated getting more in-depth instruction in searching PubMed. Second-year students have also commented to pharmacy faculty and librarians that the drug information sources they learned about proved useful during their summer clinical practice experience. Negative comments were received from a few students who failed to understand the significance of some of the topics, especially bibliographic databases.

The do-it-yourself exercise allowed a more controlled evaluation of student understanding of online drug resources. Eighty-one assignments for this exercise were analyzed (see Table 11.3).

If the answer sheet showed that relevant information was found in the databases, it showed "some success" in locating information on a certain drug or dietary supplement. If a student mentioned the limitations of locating drug or supplement ingredient information in MEDLINE or IPA, or if comments were made about problems involved in locating information, the analysis was rated as "good." Using this rough guide to the success of the exercise, a total of fifty-five students, or 38 percent of eighty submissions, performed successful searches. Only twenty-four (44 percent) of those fifty-five students also provided a well-reasoned analysis of the problems involved in completing this assignment correctly. Of the total group of eighty students, seven made little attempt to carry out comprehensive database

TABLE 11.3. Success in locating drug information.

Student performance	# of students	% of total students
Successfully searched databases	55	67.90
Provided good analysis of problems	31	38.27
Successfully searched databases and provided good analysis of problems	24	29.63
Successfully searched databases, but provided poor analysis of problems	31	38.27
Not successful in database searches, but provided good analysis of problems	7	8.64
Not successful in database searches and provided poor analysis of problems	19	23.46
Total assignments	81	

searches. Combining this analysis with written comments, it can be concluded that many students misunderstood the objective of the exercise and spent too much time searching for a correct "answer," rather than understanding that information may not have been in the database. This assignment was offered again in 2002, with some modifications, but was deemed only moderately effective and is no longer included in the course.

CONCLUSION

Advances in computers and information technology provide new opportunities for pharmacists to expand their participation in pharmaceutical care. An acquaintance with pharmaceutical software applications, Web publishing technologies, database management, networking, and multimedia can benefit both the pharmacist and the patient. Likewise, the increasing involvement of health science librarians in informatics education demonstrates how health information professionals can play more integral roles in the health care environment.

The library's participation in this informatics course has required significant resources. In the first year, librarians received Access training and the librarian in charge of the Access lab spent considerable time developing suitable hands-on exercises to demonstrate the basic features of the software. Similarly, the lab sessions on PubMed and other online pharmacy resources have been redesigned each year in response to changes in database content and design, and to reflect some of the most current issues relevant to the pharmacy profession. With six three-hour lab sessions scheduled for each part of the course, it was necessary to share the teaching load among as many as five librarians.

This collaboration with pharmacy faculty has proved especially fruitful, for not only do students progress to their second academic year with improved drug information skills, but the library's involvement in the teaching of the database principles and design component has resulted in a greater appreciation of the role librarians can play in informatics education. This participation will hopefully lead to further collaborations with the School of Pharmacy as the library seeks to increase its participation in other areas of the pharmacy curriculum where students need to use other bibliographic resources or tools.

NOTES

1. Godwin, H.N. "The Impact of Automation—Dispensing and Distribution (Bpp-4-3)." *FIP World Congress* 62(2002).

2. Association of American Medical Colleges. "Evaluation of Medical Information Science in Medical Education." *Journal of Medical Education* 61(1986):487-543.

3. Troiano, D. "A Primer on Pharmacy Information Systems." *Journal of Healthcare Information Management* 13(1999):41-52.

4. Scherrer, C.S. and Jacobson, S. "New Measures for New Roles: Defining and Measuring the Current Practices of Health Sciences Librarians." *Journal of the Medical Library Association* 90(April 2002):164-172.

5. Broverman, C., Kapusnik-Uner J., Shalaby, J., and Sperzel, D. "A Concept-Based Medication Vocabulary: An Essential Requirement for Pharmacy Decision Support." *Pharmacy Practice Management Quarterly* 18(1998):1-20.

Chapter 12

Building an Effective User Education Program: The Medical Librarian As Coeducator at the University of the West Indies

Ernesta Greenidge
Meerabai Gosine-Boodoo

SETTING

The University of the West Indies (UWI) Medical Sciences Library (MSL) is a small medical library, with a professional staff consisting of five librarians. In addition to the traditional functional roles in administration, technical, and user services, the librarians share responsibilities for library and information instruction, and provide direction and support for the information needs of the Faculty of Medical Sciences (FMS).

Medicine, dentistry, veterinary medicine, and pharmacy are taught at the FMS. Students are attracted from within and outside of the Caribbean. In the first year of the program, the cohort varied from 160 students to more than 200. The FMS teaching modality is hybrid, including both didactic and problem-based learning approaches.

EDUCATIONAL APPROACHES

The overall teaching goal of the MSL user education program is to promote information literacy and the effective use of information resources. The goal is achieved through both curriculum-based and elective components. Influencing factors include the FMS teaching modality, access to technology at the MSL, curricular requirements, available skills of the librarians, and faculty responsiveness to library initiatives.

Librarians are continuously challenged to provide effective instructional support for users. Faced with new information technologies, improved operating systems, and changing modes of information retrieval, library staff must find innovative ways to make sure their customers make optimal use of the information available in the library.

Over the last three decades, the transfer of skills and expertise from the librarian to the user has changed significantly. Much of the groundwork for the newer instructional programs occurred in the 1970s as librarians began to question the value and motivations of library skills instruction. This led to the development of programs that were less tool-specific and more educational in nature. In addition, the focus changed to teaching the structure of the literature, search strategies, and problem-solving techniques. The goals of information management education evolved from teaching users about library tools to teaching them effective information-seeking and information management techniques.[1]

Medical librarians at the MSL offer a range of programs and services. The subject of this case study is UWI's Information Literacy Program (ILP), an elective component within the user education program. Introduced in 1996, ILP continued initiatives undertaken by the MSL when the FMS academic program commenced in 1989. From its inception, ILP included training in the use of bibliographic databases, popular software programs, basic computing skills, and the Internet.

The following list shows the courses offered over a three-year period for academic years 1996-1997, 1997-1998, and 1998-1999:

1. *International Pharmaceutical Abstracts (IPA)*
2. *Internet Resources—Dentistry*
3. *Internet Resources—Medicine*
4. *Introduction to Computers at MSL*
5. *Introduction to Computers I*
6. *Introduction to Computers II*
7. *Introduction to Epi Info*
8. *Introduction to ProCite*

9. *Introduction to Searching the MSL Catalogue*
10. *Introduction to the Internet*
11. *Introduction to the MSL Library*
12. *MEDCARIB—Basics* [introduction to searching the database of health literature of the English-speaking Caribbean]
13. *MEDLINE—Basics*
14. *MEDLINE and IPA—Basics*
15. *Ovid MEDLINE—Advanced*
16. *PubMed* [MEDLINE on the Internet]
17. [Introduction to] *Windows 95*

The stated objective of ILP was to enable library users to utilize computer-based information resources effectively and independently. All registered library users were eligible to participate in the program, and although the intended group size was twenty persons per session, group size varied. On at least one occasion, there was only a single participant. The time allotted to each course was one and a half hours or two hours. The format was a lecture accompanied by demonstration, and hands-on practice using the available computing facilities. For both compulsory and elective programs, participants were informed before the start of the session that an evaluation questionnaire would be administered. Because of the novelty of some of the subjects taught, such as the first introductory Internet courses, training was provided for library support staff and staff at other medical libraries. These learning opportunities encouraged independent use of the facilities, thereby enhancing users' capacity for self-directed learning.

In 1997-1998, the teaching of basic library and information skills had been integrated into a first-year compulsory course in medical communication. In this way, FMS students continued to receive training in effective retrieval of information, bibliographic style, and the use of databases. The introduction of this integrated component also required a commitment of time from the same small group of librarians.

In 1999-2000, a number of factors were considered in making a decision to suspend ILP. It was felt that a critical mass of persons had been reached. Some decrease in registration numbers was noted, and an increased number of no-shows was observed. A major review of the library's computing facilities, including the installation of a local area network (LAN), was in the planning stages. It was therefore agreed that ILP would be suspended to allow for evaluation and to plan for future activities.

EVALUATION METHODS

Library measurements enable planning for emerging trends and anticipating new user needs. The results of evaluation can be used to support requests for additional resources to satisfy new service demands and to prepare staff for new roles and responsibilities.[2] In evaluating ILP, records of planning activities and documentation of the courses taught were examined to observe changes that occurred in infrastructure, approach, and participation.

The completed evaluation questionnaires provided the primary data. The questionnaire was composed of nine rating items: clarity of learning objectives, adherence to learning objectives, organization of the presentation, instructor's knowledge of topic, instructor-class interaction, quality of handouts, quality of audiovisuals, effectiveness of demonstration(s), and opportunity for hands-on practice. Three checklist items on the evaluation form included class length, pace of instruction, and hands-on practice. Space was also provided for written responses to the following: best aspects of the class, recommended changes, additional training desired, and additional comments.

These evaluation items were developed to ascertain the degree of satisfaction of each participant. Two discrepancies in the questionnaire were observed. The first was that the evaluation items "clarity of learning objectives" and "adherence to objectives" were excluded from the 1997-1998 questionnaire. The second was that the evaluation item "opportunity for hands-on practice" was excluded from some of the second semester 1997-1998 evaluation forms and from all evaluation forms administered in 1998-1999.

In reviewing the planning activities that attended the introduction of ILP, it was observed that the implementation was guided by the experience of the head (1995-1999) of the MSL and that much learning occurred among the librarians as the program progressed. Formative evaluation took place while perusing completed evaluation questionnaires and the observations of the tutors. Feedback was sought from faculty members, who were encouraged to indicate which courses they would find useful and to suggest periods best suited for scheduling courses. These assessments informed the decision-making process regarding course choices, logistics, and amendments to the evaluation questionnaire, as well as the decision to suspend the program and to engage in further evaluation.

The highest percentage of favorable ratings for effective teaching was assigned to the following courses: Internet Dentistry, *MEDLINE and IPA—Basics,* and *Introduction to Searching the MSL Catalogue.* Items that received the lowest percentage of favorable ratings included "opportunity for hands-on" and "class length." "Instructor's knowledge of topic" consistently ranked high each year.

In 1996-1997, when compared to five other variables, "opportunity for hands-on" was rated "excellent" by only 25 percent of the respondents. However, in 1997-1998 it was rated the second highest with 45 percent, preceded only by "instructor's knowledge of topic." This led to further investigation of factors affecting the "excellent" score. It was observed that in 1996-1997 out of six courses, two had fewer than twelve participants and that these were the only two courses with only excellent ratings. In that year, all courses except Windows 95 received some percentage rating of "excellent."

In 1997-1998, out of eight courses taught, three attracted fewer than twelve participants. The opportunity for hands-on practice in these courses was rated favorably. The findings suggest that participants in smaller classes show higher levels of satisfaction with hands-on practice, since the "poor" rating only appeared in courses with more than twelve participants. However, size of class does not explain the overall higher rating of "excellent" in 1997-1998. Other factors may include user interest and time spent using the available computers. In 1998-1999 the question was omitted, since in formative evaluations it was felt that without the necessary infrastructure, participants did not have sufficient opportunity for hands-on practice.

Comments appearing on the evaluation forms also supported the interpretation of the ratings. "Opportunity for hands-on practice" was consistently rated as inadequate. Table 12.1 illustrates comments elicited in the Recommended Changes section of the forms, which also highlighted the urgency for upgrading computing facilities.

Courses were ranked in order of popularity based upon voluntary attendance. The findings show that the same course *(Introduction to*

TABLE 12.1. Comments on opportunity for hands-on practice.

Year	Recommended Changes
1996-1997	Hands-on experience
	One person to a computer
	More computers
	Longer time
	More sessions
	No need for change
1997-1998	More practice time allotted
	Less information and more time for hands-on
	Install the program before class starts
	Longer time to understand the workings of the software
	Demonstration while students apply
	None needed

the Internet) was ranked as the favorite in each year: 40 percent in 1996-1997; 37 percent in 1997-1998; and 20 percent in 1998-1999.

For further analysis, the courses were categorized into four groups: (1) Use of the Internet; (2) Use of Computers; (3) Use of Databases, and (4) Use of Applications Programs. The most popular group for each of the three years was as follows: Use of Computers—48 percent in 1996-1997; Use of Databases—54 percent in 1997-1998; and Use of Databases—62 percent in 1998-1999.

The progression of user needs from using computers to using databases is significant and visible. It should be noted that only data from 1998-1999 supported this observation, since it was the only year in which all four groups of courses were taught. In 1996-1997, Use of Databases had not yet been introduced. In 1997-1998, Use of Applications Programs was omitted. The "needs of the libraries' immediate users" continue to influence the library teaching program.[3]

Evaluation instruments were incorporated into all programs, both compulsory and elective. At orientation, students currently complete a questionnaire that records their knowledge of basic computing and their perceived need for information literacy training. Although computer skills do not predict information literacy skills, the completed questionnaires provide some indication of prior knowledge of computing and facility with computers.

Students of the medical communication course complete a pre-test and a post-test that measure knowledge of library research concepts. These instruments continue to provide the data for measuring effectiveness of the program and guidelines for improvement.

FUTURE PLANS

The findings have proven to be more than encouraging. The MSL is well positioned to deepen and widen the user education program, and to reach an expanded clientele based upon the strategic objectives of the university. At the Ohio State University, it was found that a key program goal "to develop and sustain effective teaching skills . . . in a user education program"[4] was to enable librarians to be more effective in their teaching. It was clear that new librarians needed orientation both to the program and to teaching, especially practical experience learning instructional techniques, developing lesson plans, and receiving evaluative feedback.[4] In response to the high user expectations inferred by comments noted in this MSL study, the librarian must ensure that he or she has the skills to communicate and teach effectively, organize lectures and demonstrations, write instructional objectives, and handle large classes. The MSL has benefited from orientation and continued teaching support through the university's Instructional Development Unit.

Continued attention to quality demands a structured approach to the administration and management of a user education program. One model for management, discussed by Allegri, elevates "education to an 'umbrella' department, encompassing such functions as reference, online services, consultation services and microcomputer services."[5] If this model were adopted, expansion of the MSL's program would require management or coordination by one individual. This is contrary to the current team-based approach at the MSL, where librarians have shared the responsibility for teaching and coordinating the training activities on a rotational basis. Undoubtedly, additional human resources would be required. Scherrer and Jacobson recommend examination of current statistics, user needs, professional library literature, and current activities."[2] This trend has been observed at MSL and will continue.

CONCLUSION

Despite limited resources, the MSL developed a user education program and successfully introduced many users to information literacy training and particularly to the Internet, which was quite a new development at the time. MSL librarians can therefore be described as early adopters and innovators. From inception, they have been continuously engaged in the range of educational programs and services offered by other medical libraries. The FMS commenced teaching in 1989 and library orientation was provided from that early stage. Introduced in 1993, bibliographic instruction consisted of tutoring in UC10D, *Research, Reporting and Documentation,* a compulsory course. By 1994, a further step was taken when the MSL stated a position on computer and information literacy skills for students of the faculty. The position statement served as the basis for MSL's User Education Program and set the groundwork for integrating library and information skills into the curriculum in 1997. In subsequent years, the need for these skills was reinforced through the requirement for student research projects presented at annual student research days.

Successful integration of information literacy training into specific programs of the FMS has been achieved in the pharmacy and veterinary medicine programs. Through this initiative, databases and Internet resources in these subject areas are covered. These compulsory curricular offerings provide additional opportunities for the librarians to support the teaching program through integrated components, which are taught annually. Opportunities for consultations and on-demand training are also accommodated. It should be noted also that notwithstanding the decision in 1999-2000 to suspend ILP, educational programming has continued.

In 2000-2001, the librarians designed and continued to teach an information literacy component for the postgraduate diploma in family medicine and primary care. The component includes Internet resources, use of the OPAC, PubMed, and basic computing/informatics.

Librarians at the MSL are cognizant of the fact that effective development of user education programs requires a major investment of time, and that the results are enhanced by faculty support. Strategic alliances with faculty have resulted in the integration of elements of the information literacy curriculum into the formal curriculum. A significant number of library users have been successfully introduced to new technologies through library programming. With the LAN now installed and stable, additional infrastructure has enabled full Internet access and increased access to electronic resources. The challenge now is to utilize the evidence derived from the evaluation of programs that have been taught.

Librarians at the MSL have teamed with counterparts in the Campus Libraries system to prepare an online information literacy product that was tested and integrated into teaching in 2003-2004. By continuing to develop this culture of research in order to better understand, plan, and develop a program that will be more satisfying to the user, the MSL clearly recognizes the need to have a quality program that is well defined with goals, activities, and future projections accompanied by standardized instructional goals and objectives.

NOTES

1. King, David N. "Creating Educational Programs in Libraries: Introduction and Part 1—Training and Education." In *User Education in Health Sciences Libraries: A Reader,* edited by M. Sandra Wood. Binghamton, NY: The Haworth Press, 1995, 7-14.

2. Scherrer, Carol S. and Jacobson, Susan. "New Measures for New Roles: Defining and Measuring the Current Practices of Health Sciences Librarians." *Journal of the Medical Library Association* 90 (April 2002):164-172.

3. Hahn, Karla L., Martin, Nadia J., and Schwartz, Diane G. "Evaluation and Future Trends." In *Educational Services in Health Sciences Libraries,* Volume 2 of *Current Practice in Health Sciences Librarianship,* edited by Alison Bunting. Metuchen, NJ: Medical Library Association and Scarecrow Press, 1995, 107-151.

4. Tiefel, Virginia. "Developing a Teaching Effectiveness Program for Librarians: The Ohio State University Experience." In *User Education in Health Sciences Libraries: A Reader,* edited by M. Sandra Wood. Binghamton, NY: The Haworth Press, 1995, 43-52.

5. Allegri, Francesca. "Administrative Structures for Education Programs." In *User Education in Health Sciences Libraries: A Reader,* edited by M. Sandra Wood. Binghamton, NY: The Haworth Press, 1995, 35-42.

Chapter 13

Educational Programs at the New York University College of Dentistry

Luis J. Gonzalez
Van B. Afes
Christopher Evjy

SETTING

The Waldmann Memorial Library serves the faculty, students, and staff of the New York University College of Dentistry (NYUCD). The library supports the largest dental school program in the United States, with over 230 students in each class of the four-year DDS (Doctorate in Dental Surgery) program, 150 students in each class of the three-year DDS Advanced Program for international dentists, a dental hygiene program, and postgraduate programs in pediatric dentistry, prosthodontics, endodontics, implant dentistry, periodontics, oral and maxillofacial surgery, orthodontics, and advanced general dentistry. Masters programs include clinical research, biomaterials sciences, and oral biology. The school has a faculty of 800, including full-time and part-time appointees.

The Waldmann Memorial Library's print collections include more than 5,000 books and current subscriptions to more than 350 professional dental journals. As a branch of the Ehrmann Medical Library of the NYU School of Medicine and a member of the NYU Library System, the Waldmann library offers on-site and remote access to more than 5,000 full-text electronic journals and 200 electronic databases.

EDUCATIONAL APPROACHES

Over the past decade, the number of electronic information resources has grown exponentially. Information vendors and providers are continually adapting and upgrading their products. The library has been confronted with evaluating and maintaining the bibliographic searching abilities and computer skills of its patrons. This has resulted in the launching of a tutorials program to train library users in the effective use of a variety of electronic resources. The goal of these tutorials is not only to enhance the computerized literature searching skills of the college community, but also to provide dynamic, ongoing instruction to accommodate constantly transforming technologies.

With the introduction of evidence-based health care practice, a new paradigm in health care, the library was invited by the Dental Pediatrics Postgraduate Program to produce a series of lectures on the basics of evidence-based dentistry for its first-year residents. The course was developed to cover the basic principles of searching and evaluating the scientific literature utilizing the new evidence-based model.

Other challenges for the library's educational program included the introduction of a new curriculum in the fall 2000 semester and the introduction of *VitalBook*, a DVD product purchased by new students that contains all the reading materials needed during their three- or four-year program. In cooperation with the Dental Informatics Department of the college, the library was charged with the task of developing a course for first-year students of the DDS and international programs to teach them to become skilled managers of information in the dental setting. Students learn how to access and evaluate information, to use evidence in clinical decision making, and to frame the parameters of a clinical inquiry. Students gain foundation knowledge in bibliographic database searching as well as other technology-based functions that enhance dental practice activities and develop expertise in the use of the *VitalBook*.

Creating a Library Tutorials Program

Assessing the College's Needs

The library developed and conducted a needs assessment survey to evaluate and determine the current computer searching skills of the college community. The survey would also provide direction about the best methods and strategies to present the information. After survey results were tabulated, an educational program could be planned and designed to fulfill the specific training and information needs of the institution.

Survey Instrument

Dental library staff cooperated staff from the Ehrman Medical Library to create and revise the survey before e-mailing the final document to NYUCD faculty and staff. The survey was formulated to provide a better understanding of existing computer skills, current use of library resources, level of comfort with computer searching, and interest in computer search instruction. The survey asked questions in the following areas:

- Respondent status in the college (full-time faculty, part-time faculty, student, administrative staff, support staff, or other)
- Library use (once a week, more than once a week, once a month, etc.)
- Library's Web page use (one or two times per week, one or two times per month, rarely, etc.)
- Level of satisfaction with library services (1 for "excellent" to 5 for "poor")
- Self-evaluation of database searching skills (beginner, intermediate, advanced, expert)
- Interest in attending scheduled library tutorials (convenient days of the week, best time of the day, offered how often)

The survey also presented a series of topics (MEDLINE searching, how to use EndNote, introduction to the World Wide Web, introduction to HTML, etc.), and users were asked to select the subjects to be covered by the tutorials. Recipients were given the choice of returning the questionnaire via e-mail or hand delivery to the library. The survey was answered and returned by 49 percent of those that received the e-mail.

Designing and Implementing the Program

Data from the survey were compiled and analyzed to determine the needs of the institution and library users. Statistics from the reference department regarding the number and type of computer help questions answered were also used. Based on these results and the reference statistics, the library decided to cover Ovid MEDLINE searching; evidence-based health care practice searching and evaluating techniques; introduction to HTML; library electronic resources orientation; and introduction to the use of EndNote, the bibliographic management software. MEDLINE searching would be offered twice a month. The HTML and evidence-based health care classes would be offered once a month and twice a month on alternate months. The EndNote class would be offered once a month. The tutorial of the library's electronic resources would be offered once a month.

The library negotiates specific numbers of simultaneous users with each electronic database provider. An instructional or teaching password is procured for each training session so that library patrons and class participants can access databases at the same time. The number of people allowed to register per class is limited to five because of the number of computers available in the classroom and to allow time for the instructor to answer individual questions.

The library negotiated access to the NYUCD Information Technology department's computer classroom on Tuesdays and Wednesdays from noon to 2:00 p.m. to conduct the tutorials. The library acquired NetSupport School from NetSupport Inc. (Productive Computer Insights Ltd.), training software that allows the instructor to control all computers in the classroom from one central workstation. This permits attendees to see what the instructor is doing on the projection screen and simultaneously on their computer monitors. When the demonstration is over, the instructor releases the computers so that attendees can practice on their own.

All tutorials are of an introductory nature. At the end of the sessions, attendees are encouraged to explore the products by themselves following the topics covered in the class and contacting the library instructors for additional help if necessary. At the end of each class, attendees are asked to evaluate the class and to make suggestions on how the class and materials offered can be improved. Refer to Box 13.1 for the course evaluation instrument.

BOX 13.1. New York University College of Dentistry Waldmann Memorial Library Tutorial Evaluation

Please take a few moments to fill out this evaluation form. You are not required to write your name. Return this form to the instructor before leaving. Thank you for your time and feedback.

1. Did this course meet your expectations?
   □ Yes   □ No
2. Were handouts and presentations helpful in understanding the material?
   □ Yes   □ No
3. Was the pace of the sessions:
   □ Too slow   □ Too fast   □ Just right
4. Was the length of the sessions:
   □ Too short   □ Too long   □ Just right
5. Was there enough time for individual questions?
   □ Yes   □ No
6. Did you feel that the level of instruction was:
   □ Too advanced   □ Too basic   □ Just right
7. How could this tutorial be improved? _____
   _____
8. Other comments: _____
   _____

Instructor's name: _____

Date: _____ Tutorial: _____

Marketing the Program

At the beginning of every month, an institutional e-mail is sent to faculty, staff, and students announcing the schedule of classes for the current month. A brief description of classes, time and date of each class, telephone number, and Web link are provided for registration. The library also places announcements on the college's closed-circuit television system including all relevant information about classes. The library's Web page also provides users with the monthly schedule of classes with links to the electronic registration pages.

Evidence-Based Dentistry for Pediatric Dental Residents

Evidence-based medicine has been defined as the process of systematically finding, appraising, and using contemporary research as the basis for clinical practice.[1] The importance of information management skills and the advent of the evidence-based health care paradigm have created a need for medical and dental schools to emphasize evidence-based training for their first-year residents. Traditionally, medical librarians have been more involved in teaching quality searching techniques and critical appraisal skills of the biomedical literature, but the trend has been expanding to include evidence-based practice. The Pediatrics Department of NYUDC invited the Waldmann Library to present a proposal for an evidence-based dentistry (EBD) course for its first-year residents. The goal was to develop literature searching and evaluation skills in accordance with the new evidence-based principles.

Librarians conducted an evaluation of the program's journal club sessions and concluded that little emphasis had been given to literature searching skills. These resident presentations were short and superficial, with little or no reference to how the literature had been selected or the material's value or validity.

Librarians developed a proposal for a four-session course that would follow the problem-based learning format and gave it to the director of the Pediatrics Department for approval. Three of the four sessions would be one-hour PowerPoint presentation lectures. The second session would be a two-hour search demonstration class in the computer lab. The library presented a program focusing on the following:

- Evidence-based health care practice, its origins, and the reasons for its advent
- Information explosion of biomedical literature
- How to practice EBD
- Changing role of the clinician from information repository to information manager
- Different types of biomedical literature and evidence-based literature resources
- Formulating a clinical question and creating a good search strategy
- Different types of study designs and research methodologies
- Appraising the biomedical literature using statistical models

Session one covers the definition of evidence-based health care practice and a brief description of the origins of its practice; information explosion in the biomedical field and its consequences for students and physicians; the concept of lifelong learning; and how to practice evidence-based health care. The session ends with a description of evidence-based-type literature and where to find it.

In session two, the formulation of the clinical question using the Patient, Intervention, Comparison of intervention, Outcome (PICO) method is covered. The session is designed to cover the different types of research questions (therapy, prognosis, diagnosis, and etiology of harm). Emphasis is also given to the different types of research studies (randomized controlled trials, cohort studies, case control studies, etc.) and associated terms (drug therapy, blinded and double-blinded studies, true positive versus true negative, survival rate, and others) that can be used to refine literature searches.

The third and fourth sessions cover how to critically appraise the literature searches by determining validity and relevance following evidence-based principles. Concepts such as number need to treat, odds ratio, relative risk, relative risk reduction, specificity versus sensitivity, positive predictive versus negative predictive values, likelihood ratio, and other statistical terms are explained in detail.

Residents are given four clinical scenarios based on therapy, diagnosis, prognosis, and etiology of harm questions and are asked to follow evidence-based principles to search the literature for each scenario. For their final evaluation, residents submit search results including search history and strategies. In addition, they are required to write critical appraisals of their results by following the rules of validity and relevance discussed in the third and fourth sessions. The evaluation of the assignments is based on the following criteria:

- *Evaluated by the librarian:* formulation of the clinical question; use of limits, controlled vocabulary versus keyword searching, Boolean logic to combine terms; selection of appropriate evidence-based resources
- *Evaluated by the Pediatrics Department:* selection of the most relevant article from the search results; rationale for why other articles in search results were not selected; validation of decisions using the parameters discussed in sessions three and four

Designing a Class for the First-Year DDS Program

In 1997, the NYUCD Curriculum Committee began planning a curriculum revision. The improved curriculum was expected to promote evidence-based decision making, foster problem solving and critical thinking, promote lifelong learning, and recognize the role of technology in the educational process.

In 1998, the college was introduced to Vital Source Technologies, Inc. (VST), and their product *VitalBook* and recognized the potential of this resource to help revise the curriculum. This product was incorporated into the curriculum with the DDS class of 2005 and offered students the advantage of having all their textbooks and class materials for the entire four-year program on a single DVD. The College of Dentistry had many expectations for *VitalBook,* including curriculum integration and involving students and faculty with technology. Students would use computers to access all aspects of their course work and faculty would use *VitalBook* to incorporate contents of textbooks into their lectures.

As students can use *VitalBook* to search a single concept across disciplines, it allows them to conceptualize the curriculum as a whole, visually representing how concepts are found both in the clinical and basic sciences.

The library's professional staff, in cooperation with the college's Dental Informatics Department, was asked to create an introductory computer technology course to be taught as part of the new first-year curriculum. *Application of Technology in Health and Health Practice* is a two-credit immersion course that uses the framework of *VitalBook* to introduce and evaluate students on the basic database searching techniques, evidence-based health care, and PowerPoint presentation software. Students are introduced to the course objectives through a series of clinical scenarios. They learn how to identify clinical questions, answer foreground and background questions, and search relevant information resources including *VitalBook* and MEDLINE. As a final class project, each student analyzes a clinical scenario and presents findings in a PowerPoint presentation. The appendix features a detailed outline of the course.

EVALUATION METHODS

The library's tutorial programs were fully instituted in the fall 2001 semester. During the first semester, eleven tutorials were conducted for a total of twenty teaching hours. Of the total thirty-nine registrants for the classes, thirty (76 percent) actually attended. During 2002, fifty-two tutorials were offered. Of 197 people registered, 163 (83 percent) attended the sessions. Of those who registered and attended tutorials, 87 percent were faculty and 13 percent were staff.

Following high attendance rates for courses held during the fall 2001 and spring 2002 semesters, attendance for *Introduction to Evidence-Based Health Care* classes has diminished considerably, despite being offered every other month. In contrast, attendance at the EndNote tutorial has increased considerably. Faculty members have requested that additional EndNote tutorials be added to the schedule. The library also started offering *RefWorks*, Web-based bibliography management software, and offered an introductory tutorial starting during the fall 2003 semester.

The four-session Evidence-Based Health Care Practice class for the Pediatric Dentistry Residency Program began its third year in the fall 2003 semester. Feedback from the Dental Pediatrics Department was very positive and the library was asked to continue offering the classes. The library made proposals to the heads of the Orthodontics, Prosthodontics, and Endodontics departments to offer similar programs to their first-year residents. The library's proposal customizes the assignment component of the course according to the topics of each program.

Application of Technology in Health and Health Practice began its third year in the fall 2003 semester. Students and the Curriculum Committee have given highly favorable comments in both sets of evaluations, and the course is now firmly established within the DDS curriculum. It is the only course of its type in the entire curriculum of New York University, and the course directors have been approached by two other dental schools to act as consultants in the creation of similar courses at their schools.

APPENDIX: APPLICATION OF TECHNOLOGY IN HEALTH AND HEALTH PRACTICE SYLLABUS

Program: D1, Fall 1

Hours: 30

Faculty: Elise S. Eisenberg, DDS, MA, Director of Dental Informatics
Van B. Afes, MA, MS, Director of the Waldman Dental Library

Course Rules and Policies: Attendance required at each class. Grade will be derived from the following: 85 percent project(s), 15 percent attendance.

Goals: This course will help students to become skilled as managers of information in a dental setting. Students will learn how to access information and become astute about the evaluation of the information found. Students will have a better understanding of the use of evidence and information in clinical decision making and learn how to frame the parameters of a clinical inquiry. Students will gain foundation knowledge in basic Internet skills, word processing, and presentation software as well as technology-based functions that enhance the activities in dental practice. Students will develop expertise with *VitalBook* and its functions.

Objectives:

- Develop skill in using e-mail, e-mail lists, Web browsing, and Web searching
- Learn how to navigate the Intranet and a variety of Internet sites
- Understand how to use a word processor and presentation software and create a presentation
- Develop expertise with *VitalBook* and its functions
- Foundation knowledge of technology-based functions that enhance the activities in dental practice
- Identification and efficient utilization of relevant information resources, including problem solving and critical decision making, formulating a clinical question, and understanding background and foreground questions
- How to access MEDLINE and use MeSH, Boolean operators, and limit commands
- How to critically appraise the literature

Lecture Topics:

1. Introduction and problem thread—four problems that thread throughout the week. Students will be broken into four groups of ~60. Each group will have a different problem. Within this group will be smaller peer groups that will work on the problem. Problems contain a dental clinical problem with treatment options. Using the tools they learn

this week, the students will research the problems, find the evidence to help them make a clinical decision, and create a presentation discussing the problem.
2. Framing the parameters of a clinical inquiry.
3. Technology-based functions in a dental practice.
4. Evidence-based approaches to clinical decision making—information at the point of care.
5. Doing a case presentation.
6. PowerPoint overview.
7. Personal digital assistant overview.
8. Review and student presentations.

Training Topics:

Basic Computer/Internet Topics—4 hours
1. Using the Internet—Web browser, e-mail/NYUHome (2 hours)
2. Word processing basics (1 hour)
3. PowerPoint basics (1 hour)
VitalBook Training—3 hours
1. Basic usage (2 hours)
2. Advanced concepts (1 hour)
Library Training—4 hours
1. MEDLINE (2 hours)
2. Web-based searches (1 hour)
3. Other databases (1 hour)

The course is designed to fulfill the following competency requirements for graduation:

Competency/Educational Outcome: 3A

3. Access, evaluate, and apply evidence-based findings from the biomedical, social, and clinical sciences utilizing conventional and electronic informational resources as a strategy for lifelong learning, when making health care decisions.

A. The student will access appropriate literature, reference books, and other data in the care of his or her patients.

Means of Assessment: Simulation
Description of Simulation Exercise:

For the entire course:

PowerPoint class presentations of case studies, including formulation of the clinical question, answering background *(VitalBook)* and foreground (MEDLINE) questions, e-mail assignments sent to instructors, and assignments during conferences. Criteria for evaluation: checklists, in-class assignments, and presentations.

For the Information Technology Section:
  Students will be asked to complete the following exercise:

a. Send, reply, forward e-mail with attachment to other members of the group
b. Virus scan an attachment received and view it
c. Navigate through the NYUCD Intranet
d. Download files from Web sites and scan for viruses
e. Utilize plug-ins for a variety of Web sites
f. View an Adobe Acrobat file
g. Perform a search on a Web-based search engine (Yahoo, Excite, etc.)
h. Review how to create, modify, print, and save word processing documents and presentations
i. Cut and paste information from other resources into word processing documents and presentations
j. Create a PowerPoint document
k. Learn how to work with Blackboard, including on-line quiz/assessment

For the Information Resource Section:
  Students will be asked to complete the following exercise utilizing the MEDLINE database:

a. How many citations do you find on the etiology of tooth diseases?
b. Find information about the Maryland Bridge restoration technique on patients over sixty-five years old.
c. Look for information about the relation of dental implants and smoking.
d. How many studies show that the combination of flossing and brushing prevents tooth decay?
e. Find information about the antileukemia drug called "gleevec."

Evaluation Criteria:

The student, in simulation exercises, will demonstrate his or her ability to access the professional literature by:

a. developing a literature/information search strategy, and
b. executing a literature/information search and finding answers to specific questions utilizing the MEDLINE database.

The students, in groups of four to six, will demonstrate the skills learned in the course through a PowerPoint presentation based on a clinical case study.

NOTE

1. Sackett, D.L., Richardson, W.S., Rosenberg, W., and Haynes, R.B. *Evidence-Based Medicine: How to Practice and Teach EBM,* 2nd ed. New York: Churchill Livingstone, 2000.

BIBLIOGRAPHY

Bradigan, P.S. and Mularski, C.A. "End-User Searching in a Medical School Curriculum: An Evaluated Modular Approach." *Bulletin of the Medical Library Association* 77(October 1989):348-356.

Burnham, J.F. "Promoting Interaction Between Organizations of Medical Librarians and Health Care Professionals." *Bulletin of the Medical Library Association* 87(January 1999):77-80.

Burrows, S.C. and Tylman, V. "Evaluating Medical Student Searches of MEDLINE for Evidence-Based Information: Process and Application of Results." *Bulletin of the Library Medical Association* 87(October 1999):471-476.

Earl, M.F. "Library Instruction in the Medical School Curriculum: A Survey of Medical College Libraries." *Bulletin of the Medical Library Association* 84 (April 1996):191-195.

Earl, M.F. and Neutens, J.A. "Evidence-Based Medicine Training for Residents and Students at a Teaching Hospital: The Library's Role in Turning Evidence into Action." *Bulletin of the Medical Library Association* 87(April 1999):211-214.

Eldredge, J.D. "A Problem-Based Learning Curriculum in Transition: The Emerging Role of the Library." *Bulletin of the Medical Library Association* 81(July 1993):310-315.

Greenhalgh, T. *How to Read a Paper: The Basics of Evidence Based Medicine,* edited by BMJ Publishing Group. London: BMJ Publishing Group, 1997.

Hahn, K.L., Martin, N.J., and Schwartz, D.G. "Evaluation and Future Trends." In *Educational Services in Health Sciences Libraries,* Volume 2 of *Current Practice in Health Sciences Librarianship,* edited by Alison Bunting. Metuchen, NJ: Medical Library Association and Scarecrow Press, 1995, 107-151.

Lewis, M. "Library Requirements and Problem-Based Learning: The Medical Sciences Library, the University of the West Indies." *Bulletin of the Medical Library Association* 88(July 2000):255-257.

McGowan, J.J. "The Role of Health Sciences Librarians in the Teaching and Retention of the Knowledge, Skills, and Attitudes of Lifelong Learning." *Bulletin of the Medical Library Association* 83(April 1995):184-189.

Moore, M. "Innovation and Education: Unlimited Potential for the Teaching Library." *Bulletin of the Medical Library Association* 77(January 1989):26-32.

Scherrer, C.S. and Dorsch, J.L. "The Evolving Role of the Librarian in Evidence-Based Medicine." *Bulletin of the Medical Library Association* 87(July 1999): 322-328.

Chapter 14

Education Services
at the Health Sciences Library
of the University of North Carolina
at Chapel Hill

Julia Shaw-Kokot

INTRODUCTION

The Health Sciences Library (HSL) at the University of North Carolina at Chapel Hill (UNC–Chapel Hill) supports a diverse academic, state, and alumni community. The library is committed to providing innovative, high-quality educational support to these ever-changing communities. During nearly twenty-five years of instructional services, the world of health care, libraries, and the people who provide access to services in these areas have undergone many changes. The resulting information evolution from print to electronic and instant access provide both challenges and rewards for all librarians, especially those involved in education services.

SETTING

The University of North Carolina at Chapel Hill was the first state university in the United States and has educated ten generations of students. The university's mission is to serve the needs of everyone in the state. It is also a major research institution with over $438 million in contracts and grants in the fall of 2001, including $236.8 million received from the National Institutes of Health.[1]

The HSL building is situated in the middle of the unofficial Health Affairs side of campus. This location is convenient for on-campus faculty, staff, and students from the Schools of Dentistry, Medicine, Nursing, Pharmacy, and Public Health, as well as staff from the on-campus UNC Hospitals (600 beds), clinics, and other support units. Allied health schools, including Clinical Laboratory Medicine and Physical Therapy, fall under the umbrella of the School of Medicine.

The UNC–Chapel Hill campus is currently one contiguous area. However, because of academic and clinical program expansions, offices are scattered throughout the wide geographic area of Raleigh, Durham, Chapel Hill, Research Triangle Park, and other areas of the state. Plans are also underway to develop a new campus area on land several miles north of the current campus.

There are sixteen libraries on the UNC–Chapel Hill campus, including the HSL. The Academic Affairs Libraries and the Law Library work closely with the HSL to provide access to information and collaborative ventures, including collection development and electronic presence.

An active Information Technology (IT) staff provides and supports hardware, software, and the library's electronic presence and development. The library is part of a robust centrally administered campus network and works with the School of Medicine and UNC Hospitals computer support units. These external units provide all password, identification, and other user administration. The HSL IT group supports all staff and public access computers within the library building except those in the Academic Technology Network computer lab.

PARTICIPANTS

The HSL's main educational focus has always been the students, faculty, and staff of the Health Affairs schools and UNC Hospitals. This group includes undergraduate, professional, and graduate students and those seeking special certification or other program recognition. University research is supported by a large number of post-doctoral staff. The clinical nature of health affairs schools allows for a large number of adjunct and clinical faculty, and the hospitals offer programs for all levels of health care workers including residency and fellowship programs for medical house staff.

The library also serves the central office of the North Carolina Area Health Education Centers (AHECs), located on the UNC campus, and as the primary resource library for six AHEC libraries and their associated health care sites. The AHEC libraries are spread throughout the state and serve a variety of health care sites, including hospitals, public health departments, clinics, and physician offices. Many off-campus preceptors are affiliated with and supported by both AHEC and UNC-Chapel Hill.

The HSL also works with student, faculty, and staff from the entire university. In 2001, the total university population included 25,480 students and 2,600 full-time faculty members.[1] Education librarians serve on campuswide groups that provide training and support for university faculty and teaching assistants. Along this line, the library is also actively involved with the School of Information and Library Science and librarians serve as adjunct faculty, guest lecturers, grant collaborators, and mentors for students.

The UNC–Chapel Hill campus has offered off-site degree and continuing education programs for many years with AHEC libraries that support Health Affairs off-campus programs. Currently, the Library supports students from around the world who are enrolled in one of the many distance education courses. Education Services staff also work with medical and nursing alumni.

Since the university's stated mission is to support the entire state, the library offers regular sessions for public and community college librarians through a contract with the State Library of North Carolina and through development programs for the public health nurses. The library also provides NC Health Info links for MEDLINEplus to give information on finding health care throughout the state.

EDUCATIONAL APPROACHES

The HSL's Education Services (ES) group is part of the User Services Department and consists of three full-time equivalent librarians including the education services coordinator, a curriculum support specialist who is an instructional designer, a twenty-hour-per-week library school student, a half-time clinical pediatrics librarian, a database support specialist, and the reserves manager. Although many library staff members provide instruction in special areas, user education is usually coordinated by the ES group. Keys to the library's educational programs are perseverance, creativity, teamwork, and publicity (see Figure 14.1). Box 14.1 provides more information about program management aspects.

To support such a widespread and diverse user population, library staff identified a list of core information competencies (see Appendix) that are used to plan and design instructional sessions. These "draft" competencies are reviewed and changed to incorporate new competencies as needed. This document has opened doors and provided opportunities as the library's user groups have focused increas-

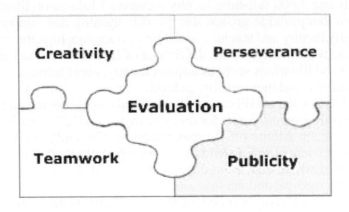

FIGURE 14.1. Program management.

BOX 14.1. Program Aspects

Perseverance
- Keep trying
- Work in small steps instead of big leaps
- Set goals and directions, but be flexible

Teamwork
- Involve everyone from faculty to students
- Identify the best people to accomplish the project

Creativity
- Brainstorm—no idea is too crazy to consider
- Know the trends
- Constantly update

Publicity
- Word of mouth is very important
- Use all avenues available
- Be seen and speak up

ingly on case- and evidence-based practice, outcome measures, and competency testing.[2]

The competencies emphasize (1) assisting in the development of information literacy competencies; (2) creating and managing personal databases using standard bibliographic formatting software; and (3) referring to and using relevant information resources in courses, tutorials, presentations, or Web pages. These competencies are based on the Medical Informatics Objectives prepared by the Association of American Medical Colleges (AAMC). AAMC's model uses a broad rather than detailed approach.[3]

When considering topics, ES staff focus on information literacy concepts rather than computer skills such as using e-mail or specific office productivity software. Users interested in learning computer skills are referred to the campus computing center. However, because the computing center classes are offered on the other side of campus, making it difficult for hospital personnel to attend, computing classes have also been offered by the computing center's training staff in the library's computer classroom.

From 2002 to 2005, renovation processes left the library without any classrooms or computer lab spaces for thirty months. Prior to renovation, there was one computer laboratory classroom that also served as an open lab for courseware. A discussion of postrenovation teaching facilities will follow under Future Plans. However, having an in-house facility supported by library staff has been most beneficial.

ES programs use a wide variety of instructional techniques that include face-to-face classes, developing Web-based modules and documentation that can be incorporated in course pages, electronic reserves, and online course assignments. Over the years, the delivery method has evolved to reflect the changing needs. There is no one-size-fits-all approach. Table 14.1 presents an overview of the identified advantages and disadvantages of the library's major instructional delivery methods.

One significant move has been toward more curriculum-integrated classes and fewer open classes. Open classes are presented on a regular basis with users registering to attend. These classes provide a way to showcase new hot topics, but in the age of ubiquitous electronic access, a big hook is needed to get busy people to attend classes. Currently, mobile technologies are of interest to many people, and the li-

TABLE 14.1. Comparison of teaching methods.

Teaching methods	Advantages	Disadvantages
Open classes	• Standard outline/format • Little preparation after initial testing/presentation • Once set, numerous instructors can follow format	• More staff time required to schedule, register, etc. • Unknown audience with different skill levels and interests
Course integrated classes	• Commitment/endorsement by faculty • Instruction related to other assignments and not seen as an "add on" • Clearly defined goals and objectives • Known group • Faculty feedback • Opportunity for evaluation	• Each class is customized • Increased time commitment • Faculty and library goals can differ
Electronic instruction	• Always available • Built-in feedback • Accommodates different learning styles • Allows for collaboration and sharing	• Time intensive • Frequent updating • Access and software issues

brary sponsors regular open forums related to personal digital assistants (PDAs). These will continue as long as attendance and interest remain high. ES still offers open classes on bibliographic formatting software and attendance continues to grow.

Recognition of the advantages of curriculum-integrated classes has been presented in the literature.[4-5] Librarians are key team members for planning, developing, teaching, and evaluating the *Pre-Clinical Information Course* and a case-based breast cancer session offered in the first-year School of Medicine curriculum. ES staff work with faculty in all areas to provide this type of instruction. For example, the librarian representative to the dental school designed, organized, and taught sessions in an information-intensive course for second-year students. In the 2001-2002 school year, 63 percent of ES courses were course-integrated.

Both open and course-integrated classes can be offered in face-to-face or electronic formats using videoconferencing and streaming video. ES staff members have also experimented with using the Library Systems and Services, Inc. (LSSI)'s meeting room feature and the telephone for distance education classes. The drawback to all these approaches is that the class has to meet together, and with students around the world this is not possible.

In 1996, ES staff received special university funding to develop six online tutorials.[6] The success of these tutorials has led to the development of many more. The primary goal of online instruction development is to produce tools that can be used when and where needed. With this in mind, the modules are Web-based and easy for faculty to link to from either HTML-developed course pages or through course management systems such as Blackboard. This approach provides seamless access to course materials including electronic reserves. Many of these modules have evaluation forms that allow the user to e-mail the completed information. The HSL Learning Modules <http://www.hsl.unc.edu/services/learning.cfm> are located on the library's Web site.

A unique collaboration with *English 12* instructors has developed as a result of faculty concerns about the quality of writing skills for students entering Health Affairs schools. *English 12* instructors are teaching assistants with little or no experience teaching, finding health information, or helping freshmen find this information. Working with these instructors over a period of several years, ES staff members have developed a two-prong approach. A basic Web-based module <http://www.hsl.nc.edu/lm/fhi/index.htm> is used to teach the students how to use health resources to find information. Course-integrated sessions assist the students in using the information presented in the module. Feedback from students and instructors has been very positive, and the module is now being used for new students in the Health Affairs schools. As the first *English 12* students enter these schools, there are anecdotal reports that the program is worthwhile.

The library developed a Media Kitchen to support users needing to work with various media, design presentations, or develop Web pages.[7] This facility allowed library staff to work one-on-one with users creating these products. Hospital house staff preparing presentations were frequent users of the facility. They could scan images from journals and incorporate them into PowerPoint presentations during off times and still be close enough to the hospital to return when called. This service was placed on hold during the library renovation.

EVALUATION METHODS

The ES mantra is to evaluate everything continuously, make changes based on evaluation, and realize that some approaches are going to fail. Growth depends on experimentation, and although not all experiments are successful, they can serve as learning experiences for future endeavors. Along with this, it must be understood that there can be no sacred cows. This a difficult hurdle at times because certain things have been held as givens. However, if a statistical and evaluation review shows that something is not working, and revamping has not improved the measures of success, it is time to end the program or change the delivery.

Providing open library orientations is an example of a program that ended due to these factors. Previously, open orientations were scheduled at the beginning of each semester in the hope of reaching new people on campus. They worked well—so well, in fact, that instructors were assigning groups of as many as sixty students to come to an open orientation. The library's classroom could handle about twenty-five people. Instructors were angry that their students did not get an orientation, students were angry that they could not get into the orientation that was on their schedule, and the library staff was frustrated. Open orientations were discontinued. Instructors now schedule orientations for their classes, and satisfaction levels have greatly increased for all involved.

The big questions related to evaluation include identifying measurement opportunities, defining reasonable outcome measures that reflect competencies, and knowing if skills are used after graduation. ES struggles with these questions and has not developed all the answers. Working with faculty in integrating library education into classes is beginning to pay off in providing measurement opportunities. For example, assisting with the integration of PDAs into the School of Nursing curriculum has yielded data on information use and information-seeking skills. Online assignments for pharmacy and dental students allow the comparison of their responses to "identified" best answers.

FUTURE PLANS

ES plans include integrating and expanding services within the renovated library space. The new facility will feature two classrooms, a videoconference room, an advanced technology center, and more Media Kitchens. Planning for these facilities has allowed the opportunity to look at use and target audiences.

Staff members are working with the campus computing center to develop video applications to enhance the online presence. With the recent addition of a new librarian, ES will be more closely involved with bioinformatics programs on campus. Collaboration with all areas of campus informatics programs is growing, and staff are involved in the planning and delivery of an interdisciplinary Health Affairs Web-based informatics course.

Other efforts include measuring nurses' postgraduation use of PDAs and other information; following pediatrics house staff information skills throughout their time at the hospitals; and comparing past *English 12* students with those who placed out of the course or transferred from another institution. As always, the staff members look at trends and hot new issues that can be incorporated into education offerings.

The future is promising, and ES staff plans to build on established relationships and develop new partnerships that will allow all participants to develop the information-seeking knowledge and skills necessary to be better health care providers, informed consumers, and healthier people. This is a big goal, but one that the library has committed to reaching.

APPENDIX:
CORE INFORMATION LITERACY COMPETENCIES

The Health Sciences Library's Education Services group is committed to working with faculty and students to determine which information literacy competencies students should demonstrate before graduating from one of the five Health Affairs schools at UNC–Chapel Hill, and to developing effective means for teaching the identified skills.

Integration of these competencies into the curriculum gives them relevance and validity. It allows the student to use the skills as part of required learning activities that can be transferred from one setting, the university, to another, the profession.

There are several ways to define core skills or competencies. Many groups, such as the American College of Preventive Medicine and other libraries, identify core competencies as discrete tasks.

The main problem with this approach is the need for constant revision. We based our thinking on the *Medical Informatics Objectives Project* prepared by the Association of American Medical Colleges (AAMC) <http://www.aamc.org/meded/msop/starthtm>, which look at broader concepts.

Since tasks are concrete activities used to practice and demonstrate the learning of concepts, it is necessary to identify specific tasks related to the broader competencies and incorporate them into the learning objectives of specific curricula.

The AAMC Medical Informatics Advisory Panel considered what roles the competencies would support and identified the following:

1. Lifelong learner
2. Clinician
3. Educator/communicator
4. Researcher
5. Manager

We feel that these are the roles most of our graduates will fill to some extent. For our purposes, we use the term *professional* for *clinician.* It seems that most competencies are necessary for all areas.

Graduate's Role

1. Demonstrate the ability to identify and express an information need and plan a search strategy to meet it, by:
   a. Clearly articulating the question or issue
   b. Outlining an action plan
   c. Identifying how the information will be used:
      • Research
      • Decision making (patient care, community needs, etc.)
      • Consumer education

2. Demonstrate knowledge about information resources relevant to the field by:
   a. Identifying key print and electronic resources
      - Textbooks and reference sources
      - Databases (bibliographic and full-text)
      - Internet sites
      - Journals
      - Accessing and retrieving information from on and off campus using relevant resources such as:
        Online catalogs
        UNCLE
        Internet
   b. Selecting, filtering, evaluating, and reconciling information on a topic by:
      - Identifying the factors that influence the accuracy and validity of information
      - Discriminating among types of information sources in terms of
        currency
        format
        authority
        relevance
        availability
      - Using multiple information sources
3. Exhibit good information skills by:
   a. "Maintaining a healthy skepticism about the quality and validity of all information" (AAMC)
   b. "Making decisions based on evidence, when such is available, rather than opinion" (AAMC)
   c. Being aware of and correctly applying copyright and intellectual property guidelines and regulations
   d. Adapting to the ever-changing skills needed for information management
4. Create and manage a personal database using standard bibliographic formatting software, including:
   a. Downloading information from a database or Web site
   b. Entering information not available by downloading
   c. Using the information to create papers and bibliographies
5. Refer to and use relevant information resources in courses, tutorials, or information pages by:
   a. Identifying and selecting appropriate print and electronic resources
   b. Using Web tools to incorporate excerpts from or links to information resources

HSL's Role

1. Work with faculty and student by providing:
   a. Instruction based on sound educational principles
   b. One-on-one assistance in person, electronically, or using other appropriate methods
   c. Organized course-integrated sessions with feedback to students and faculty
   d. Web-based online modules, links to resources and instructional materials, or other relevant tools for general or course-specific purposes
   e. Transition skills between the academic and practice settings
2. Evaluation
   a. Observation of student behavior
   b. Direct feedback to and from students and faculty
   c. Testing mechanisms
   d. Indications that alumni are using these skills

School's Role

1. Work with librarians to build information competencies; adopt core information competencies
2. Provide opportunities for accomplishing the competencies within existing curricula
3. Require demonstrated evidence of achievement of the competencies by time of graduation
4. Promote the value of attaining these competencies as part of being a successful health professional

NOTES

1. "UNC-Chapel Hill: Quick Facts About Carolina." Available: <http://www.unc.edu/depts/design/quickfacts/>.

2. Moore, M.E. and Shaw-Kokot, J. "Core Competencies." *Medical Reference Services Quarterly* 19(Winter 2000):99-103.

3. Association of American Medical Colleges. *Learning Objectives for Medical Student Education: Guidelines for Medical Schools.* Washington, DC: Association of American Medical Colleges, 1998. Available <http:www.aame.org/meded/msop/msop1.pdf>.

4. Tennant, M.R. and Miyamoto, M.M. "The Role of Medical Libraries in Undergraduate Education: A Case Study in Genetics." *Journal of the Medical Library Association* 90(April 2002):181-193.

5. Finkel, M.L., Brown, H.A., Gerber, L.M., and Supino, P.G. "Teaching Evidence-Based Medicine to Medical Students." *Medical Teacher* 25(March 2003): 202-204.

6. Loven, B., Morgan, K., Shaw-Kokot, J., and Eades, L. "Information Skills for Distance Learning." *Medical Reference Service Quarterly* 17(Fall 1998):71-75.

7. Ladd, R. "Food for Thought: Recipes for the New Century." *Medical Reference Service Quarterly* 19(Fall 2000):89-93.

Chapter 15

A Month-Long Daily Instruction Curriculum for Residents at the University of Pittsburgh: Can Intensive Training Make a Difference?

Nancy Tannery
Mark L. Scheuer
Jill E. Foust
Patricia Weiss Friedman
Amy L. Gregg
Ammon S. Ripple

INTRODUCTION

Medicine is evolving at a rapidly increasing pace. Keeping current with accurate, up-to-date, evidence-based information has become complicated and time consuming. One study examined a group of internal medicine residents' clinical encounters.[1] It found that two new questions arose for every three patients seen in clinical settings. However, residents pursued answers for only 29 percent of the new questions they encountered. Lack of time was listed as one of the reasons for these unanswered questions.

A study of family physicians found that they did not pursue answers to most of their questions, and when they did look for answers the time spent was less than two minutes.[2] Colleagues and print texts provided the sources for the majority of the answers pursued. Electronic resources were used only 2 percent of the time, and the physicians spent over six minutes searching with minimum success.

A review article in the BMJ states that information needs do arise during patient encounters.[3] Clinicians could find the answers to their questions through electronic resources but lack the skill to do so.

The utilization of immediately available electronic information resources might provide an efficient and effective method for locating evidence-based medicine information. Previous studies have described a variety of methods to provide clinicians with the information skills to use these electronic information resources. One-time workshop sessions have been described that were divided into didactic and hands-on instructional sessions on MEDLINE.[4] Other studies discuss freestanding curricula that offer workshops for one to two hours over several weeks,[5] or across several months.[6-7] Integrated evidence-based medicine training in established curricula such as journal clubs, morning reports, and attending rounds has also been explored.[8-10]

The University of Pittsburgh's month-long pilot training program for residents utilizes available electronic resources to efficiently locate answers to clinical questions. The objective of the program is to teach residents the information skills necessary to answer questions seen in patient care settings.

SETTING

The University of Pittsburgh Health Sciences Library System (HSLS) provides collections and services to meet the information needs of the educational, clinical, and research programs of the Schools of Medicine, Dental Medicine, Pharmacy, Health and Rehabilitation Sciences, Nursing, and the Graduate School of Public Health, as well as the hospitals of the University of Pittsburgh Medical Center. The HSLS electronic collection offers on-site and remote access to approximately thirty Web-based databases and full-text resources. The collection also offers access to over 2,000 electronic journals and 600 electronic books. Reference librarians provide instruction on an open-registration basis as well as through the curricula of the schools of the health sciences. The HSLS roster of classes has expanded to nineteen courses including orientation sessions and seminars on clinical, mental health, and basic sciences resources as well as bibliographic management tools, software training, and the Internet.

The Department of Neurology at the University of Pittsburgh offers a four-year training program to new medical school graduates, or a three-year training program to candidates who have successfully completed one year of postgraduate medical training. Residents and, electively, senior residents begin their first year with Intensive Introduction to Clinical Neurology, a full time, one-month course. Residents participate in case simulations and rehearsals, an intensive clinical neuropharmacology lecture series, a series of interactive neuroradiology-neuroanatomy correlation sessions, and neurological examination rounds.

A hands-on medical information retrieval segment using extensive electronic medical databases and resources is also a part of this introductory course. The course represents a collaboration between HSLS and the graduate medical education director of the neurology department. This case study describes the participation of five first-year neurology residents and a third-year chief resident in this intensive multifaceted training, with five reference librarians alternating as instructors and providing daily, individualized interactions with the residents.

EDUCATIONAL APPROACHES

Initially, the residents were presented with a brief introduction to electronic information resources and how to access them. The introduction demonstrated the HSLS Web page that provided links to PubMed, Ovid MEDLINE, evidence-based medicine databases (Clinical Evidence and the Cochrane Database of Systematic Reviews), MICROMEDEX, MD Consult, UpToDate, and electronic journal and book collections. The American Academy of Neurology practice guidelines Web site was also shown. A ninety-minute pre-test was administered after the introduction and prior to further instruction.

Residents spent one to two hours per day for twenty-one days in structured, intensive sessions related to the use of electronic information resources. This first part of the training included librarian-led interactive instruction in the effective use of the available resources. The first two sessions were spent on MEDLINE searching, using both Ovid MEDLINE and PubMed. Instruction focused on structuring a search and critically appraising the results. During the third session, residents practiced their MEDLINE skills by answering a series of clinical questions. A reference librarian provided individual feedback on search strategy and retrieval. Four sessions were allotted to instruction on evidence-based medicine theory and information resources. Overviews of PITTCat, MICROMEDEX, MD Consult, and UpToDate followed. Librarian participation in these training sessions is an extension of the HSLS instructional programs. Librarians adapted or customized regular class content for the neurology residents.

The second half of the program focused on sharpening the skills learned. Residents practiced their skills by answering questions pertinent to cases presented on that day's morning report or questions from the residency director. Each resident worked at an individual computer workstation within the library. Reference librarians and the residency director provided close, focused support. At the conclusion of the course, a ninety-minute post-test, similar in construction to the pre-test, was administered.

EVALUATION METHODS

On the section asking the residents to state the end result or the answer to the question, first-year residents achieved a mean score of 6.1/10 on the pre-test, and 7.7/10 on the post-test ($p = 0.01$, two-tailed paired t-test). This represented a mean improvement of 29 percent over their initial performance. In general, substantial improvements were evident in the choice of appropriate resources to answer specific questions. Only two of the six residents demonstrated improvement on articulating structural clinical questions. The chief resident, who had received prior training that overlapped with the course's content, performed well on both the pre- and post-test.

The pre- and post-tests consisted of five clinical scenarios that raised specific questions. An example of a post-test is included in Box 15.1. Four of the scenarios were treatment questions and one was a drug interaction question. For each scenario, the residents were required to define the clinical problem, list the resources or databases used to locate the answer, and state the end result or the answer to the question, including supporting references. Two points were assigned to each of these three parts, with a total of six points for each scenario. Each test totaled thirty points. A reference librarian and the residency

---

BOX 15.1. Neurology Residents Post-test

1. Are antidepressants, such as amitriptyline, effective treatments for migraine headaches as compared to other drugs that might be used such as beta blockers or anticonvulsants?
   What is the problem? _____
   Resources or databases used? _____
   End result? _____
2. A previously healthy thirty-year-old developed moderately severe Guillain-Barré syndrome. You are asked whether recent data favor intravenous immunoglobulin therapy or plasmapheresis as the treatment of choice. What is your response?
   What is the problem? _____
   Resources or databases used? _____
   End result? _____
3. A seventeen-year-old girl recently began having complex partial seizures. A brain MRI demonstrated findings consistent with left mesial temporal sclerosis. She initially received treatment with phenytoin and her seizures were better, but not completely controlled. She has developed hirsutism and some coarsening of her skin. The medical intern on the service suggested switching the patient's therapy to lamotrigine, stating that she had been told by one of the attending neurologists that this drug had a favorable side effect profile and was an effective antiseizure drug. The service attending stated that he was not certain about lamotrigine's effectiveness as monotherapy and wondered whether there was evidence that lamotrigine was as effective as an antiseizure agent as carbamazepine. Please answer these questions.
   What is the problem? _____
   Resources or databases used? _____
   End result? _____
4. A thirty-five-year-old woman with a history of complex partial seizures developed bronchitis. Her epilepsy was well-controlled on carbamazepine monotherapy. She was taking carbamazepine 400 mg bid and was given erythromycin and Robitussin DM for treatment of the bronchitis. Two days later she called the neurology clinic, complaining of a severe sensation of lightheadedness, double vision, and unsteadiness of gait. Could an adverse drug interaction be contributing to the patient's symptoms? If so, which drugs might be interacting to cause this constellation of symptoms?
   What is the problem? _____
   Resources or databases used? _____
   End result? _____
5. For patients with Bell's palsy, which is more effective in improving facial function outcomes, steroids or no treatment?
   What is the problem? _____
   Resources or databases used? _____
   End result? _____

director separately graded the tests. Results of the pre- and post-tests were compared.

Six months after the completion of the training course, residents completed a brief survey to assess the long-term effects of the course. Residents were asked four questions and asked to use a five-point scale to rate their abilities in four skill areas:

- Recognizing patient problems and construct a structured clinical question
- Searching the medical literature to retrieve an evidence-based answer
- Critically appraising the evidence gathered
- Using the evidence to provide the best care to their patients

The response choices were much better, better, no change, worse, and much worse, relative to their abilities before the training course. The results of the self-assessment survey completed six months after training demonstrated that the residents felt better and much better about the skills they had learned. The results suggest that the residents felt their ability to recognize patient problems, search the medical literature, critically appraise the results, and use the evidence to provide better patient care increased because of the training course.

CONCLUSION

This study indicates that providing novice neurology residents with intensive training in the effective use of information resources significantly improves their self-perceived ability to find and assess information regarding the diagnosis and treatment of neurological disorders. The results also suggest that more in-depth instruction in one skill area, constructing a structured clinical question, is necessary.

Limitations of the study include the small number of participants, the lack of a control group, and the fact that evaluations were not blinded to either the residency director or the reference librarian who graded them.

The training model described here could be adapted for other resident populations. Ideally, intensive training in the effective use of information resources started early in residency training can promote better lifelong self-directed learning. Additional studies to assess the impact of this type of intense training are warranted, especially related to the durability of acquired skills, and whether follow-up sessions should be added in the second and third years of training. Future work is needed to investigate the possibility of other positive changes such as finding and using information at the point of care and in the quality of care itself.

NOTES

1. Green, Michael L., Ciampi, Marc A., and Ellis, Peter J. "Residents' Medical Information Needs in Clinic: Are They Being Met?" *American Journal of Medicine* 109(August 2000):218-223.

2. Ely, John W., Osheroff, Jerome A., Ebell, Mark H., Bergus, George R., Levy, Barcey T., Chambliss, M. Lee, and Evans, Eric R. "Analysis of Questions Asked by Family Doctors Regarding Patient Care." *BMJ* 319(August 1999):358-361.

3. Smith, Richard. "What Clinical Information Do Doctors Need?" *BMJ* 313 (October 1996):1062-1068.

4. Bradley, Doreen R, Rana, Gurpreet K., Martin, Patricia W., and Schumacher, Robert E. "Real-Time, Evidence-Based Medicine Instruction: A Randomized Controlled Trial in a Neonatal Intensive Care Unit." *Journal of the Medical Library Association* 90(April 2002):194-201.

5. Smith, Christopher A., Ganschow, Pamela S., Reilly, Brendan M., Evans, Arthur T., McNutt, Robert A., Osei, Albert, Saquib, Muhammad, Surabhi, Surabhi, and Yadav, Sunil. "Teaching Residents Evidence-Based Medicine Skills: A Controlled Trial of Effectiveness and Assessment of Durability." *Journal of General Internal Medicine* 15(October 2000):710-715.

6. Ross, Robert, and Verdieck, Alex. "Introducing an Evidence-Based Medicine Curriculum into a Family Practice Residency—Is It Effective?" *Academic Medicine* 78(April 2003):412-417.

7. Evans, Michael. "Creating Knowledge Management Skills in Primary Care Residents: A Description of a New Pathway to Evidence-Based Practice." *ACP Journal Club* 135(September/October 2001):A11-A12.

8. Edwards, Karen S., Woolf, Paul K., and Hetzler, Theresa. "Pediatric Residents As Learners and Teachers of Evidence-Based Medicine." *Academic Medicine* 77(July 2002):748.

9. Green, Michael L. "Evidence-Based Medicine Training in Graduate Medical Education: Past, Present and Future." *Journal of Evaluation in Clinical Practice* 6(May 2000):121-138.

10. Green, Michael L. "Evidence-Based Medicine Training in Internal Medicine Residency Programs: A National Survey." *Journal of General Internal Medicine* 15(February 2000):129-133.

Chapter 16

Health Care Informatics Education at Stony Brook University: Evolution of End User Education and Mission Redefinition for the Academic Health Sciences Library

Guillaume Van Moorsel

INTRODUCTION

Health care informatics concerns the theory and practice of patient-centered information management. The burgeoning growth of clinical knowledge and steady advance of technology require that health professionals command effective information management skills. Changes in clinical education have witnessed the introduction of computer-aided instruction and distance learning, growth of problem-based learning, and emphasis on evidence-based practice. Proficiency with information technology is indispensable to the health professional in training. Efforts to define a core curriculum for allied health professions emphasize the central importance of information technology training.[1] Professional organizations of occupational, physical, and respiratory therapists now require informatics training in accredited education programs.[2-4]

Satisfying these new requirements present challenges for academic programs. Even though the importance of informatics approaches self-evidence, resource constraints determine program response. Ubiquitous budget and faculty resource limitations may prevent administrators from implementing the infrastructure and knowledge resources needed to develop and sustain credible informatics training. Such compound challenges allow health sciences librarians to secure vital new roles in the educational mission of their parent institutions.

Since the mid-1990s, academic health sciences libraries across the United States and Canada have expanded their education services programs. This trend is partly in response to demands resulting from aforementioned changes in clinical education. Advantages offered by computer-aided instruction, problem-based learning, and evidence-based practice can only be leveraged from a solid understanding of information technology. Correspondingly, many traditional bibliographic instruction series have evolved into sophisticated clinical information management training programs. As of 2002, 95 percent of member libraries of the Association of Academic Health Sciences Libraries (AAHSL) had implemented education programs.[5] The library's role as educator has grown as demand for traditional library services (e.g., reference services) has sharply declined. Because users are physically able to conduct their own research without setting-foot inside the library proper, they may perceive abridged need for information mediation by librarians.

Moreover, because users enjoy increasingly seamless access to electronic resources, technical services provided by libraries have become transparent and the resources libraries must devote to the provision and support of electronic access tend to go unnoticed. Out of sight, out of mind may cause libraries to become victims of their own success. Education programs mitigate this phenomenon by providing a high-profile venue for libraries to demonstrate and raise awareness of the resources and expertise they provide. National trends in concurrent declines in reference service demand and increases in demand for education services have been amplified at Stony Brook University (SBU) (see Figure 16.1).

SETTING

At SBU, the Health Sciences Center (HSC) Library aggressively pursued these opportunities by launching a technology-based education program and planning curriculum integration. Demonstrated program effectiveness resulted in the 2001 formation of the Center for Healthcare Informatics Education (CHIE), a library-based unit

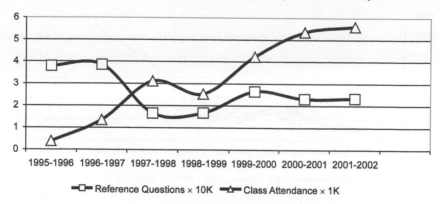

FIGURE 16.1. Education services versus information services demand.

charged with integrating informatics training into the curricula of the five professional schools of the HSC.

The HSC Library serves the academic and research missions of the Health Sciences Center, a comprehensive academic medical and health care center comprising the Schools of Dental Medicine, Medicine, Nursing, Health Technology and Management (Allied Health), and Social Welfare. Undergraduate, graduate, and postgraduate students enrolled in various health sciences programs number approximately 2,500. Each year, approximately 175 undergraduate students enter the Occupational Therapy (OT), Physical Therapy (PT), Respiratory Therapy (RT), and Physician Assistant (PA) programs.

EDUCATIONAL APPROACHES

Prior to the creation of the HSC Library's Education Services Department in 1996, user education consisted of informal bibliographic instruction workshops with little to no curricular integration. The program ranked within the fourth quartile among AAHSL members.[6]

As indicated by the growth shown in Figure 16.2, the program quickly became one of the most active in the nation. By 2000-2001, SBU ranked among the top five AAHSL programs according to all categories of measure.[5]

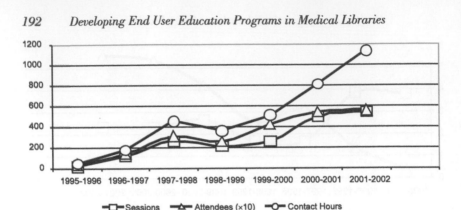

FIGURE 16.2. Educational services program growth.

Instructional offerings included database searching and information resources, desktop applications, Web development, database design, systems analysis, and information and communication systems management. Evidence-based practice courses were also offered, including research design, statistical analysis, and critical appraisal.

Curriculum Integration

By 2001-2002, HSC Library's education efforts were geared largely toward curriculum-integrated instruction. Initially, such instruction involved librarians collaborating with clinical faculty to introduce informatics lectures as a component of existing courses. In those cases, the faculty member retained primary responsibility for the parent course and its content, while the librarian assumed control for some smaller portion of the class. In some instances, librarians were responsible for up to 50 percent of the overall course.

Gibson and Silverberg have described how such a librarian-academician partnership resulted in an informatics course for medical students at SBU.[7] That success resulted in further collaborations, especially with allied health programs. Throughout the late 1990s, hundreds of library-sponsored informatics classes were offered to allied health sciences students, and demand was growing. Such growth created the following problems:

- *Inundation:* Limited size of the education department placed heavy obligations on individual librarians.
- *Fragmentation:* Offered on a class-by-class basis, piecemeal informatics instruction was not conducive to achieving desired outcomes; the combined discontinuity of instruction and lack of a "critical content mass" placed learners at a disadvantage.
- *Redundancy:* Absence of continuity in informatics instruction resulted in redundant coverage of foundational content and resistance to that content by time-sensitive learners.

Modular Course Development

To achieve the goal of educating health care professionals to be information literate, the HSC Library pursued a dual strategy. First, a systematic and standardized approach to program development was implemented. Individual workshops were developed in accordance with information literacy competencies established by the SUNY Council of Library Directors Information Literacy Initiative Committee (see Table 16.1). New ninety-minute classes were designed to be sequenced into entire programs, in which modular classes or "content blocks" can be strung together to form a foundation (see Figure 16.3). Course platforms provided a uniform foundation and boilerplate versions of support materials were used for efficient production. The system also allowed for simple modification to accommodate discipline-specific content.

Second, a similarly systematic approach was taken to cross-train all librarian-educators to teach the same content in a standardized manner. The idea of individual ownership of a given class was changed to a team approach. The result was efficient and flexible utilization of resources.

By 1999, the HSC Library argued for the need of a foundational informatics program for allied health sciences. The program started in the summer of 1999 as a required, noncredit course for all incoming OT, PT, RT, and PA students. Learner objectives included:

- to recognize the need for information;
- to understand how to access information from appropriate sources;
- to exercise best practices for integrating information into clinical decision making;

TABLE 16.1. SUNY Council of Library Directors Information Literacy Initiative Committee—information literacy core competencies.

Competency areas	Critical learning objectives and skills indicators	Cluster
Competency 1: To recognize the need for information	• Acquires conceptual understanding of the character, dimensions, and impact of the information environment	A,C
	• Learns to formulate appropriate research and information-seeking questions	
	• Incorporates effective information management into learning processes and workflow methodologies	
Competency 2: To access information from appropriate sources	• Understands nature, format, usage, benefits, and limitations of a wide variety of information resources and formats	A,B,C
	• Differentiates accuracy, coverage, currency, and intended/appropriate purpose of information resources	
	• Knows how/when to approach experts or consult guides for assistance	
Competency 3: To develop skills in using information	• Recognizes need and means of integrating accurate and timely information with technical and subject expertise	B,C
	• Exercises effective information management practices	
	• Understands principles of information mining and gathering competitive intelligence	
Competency 4: To critically analyze and evaluate information	• Adapts information evaluation skills from print-based to electronic-based environment	A,B
	• Learns new skills, methods, tools, and techniques for evaluating and filtering electronic information	
	• Appreciates the variability and uneven nature of available information in terms of accuracy and authority	
Competency 5: To organize and process information	• Learns standards for organization, classification, access, and retrieval of information in a variety of formats	A,B
	• Executes effective information searching strategies and practices efficient information resource management	
	• Uses advanced tools for access, storage, retrieval, and synthesis of information	

Competency 6: To apply information for effective decision making	• Recognizes value and importance of using information technology to support decision making	A,C
	• Undertakes appropriate action based on informed decision making	
	• Integrates individual experience and expertise with best available information and evidence	
Competency 7: To generate and communicate information and knowledge	• Understands principles of converting information into knowledge	A,B,C
	• Understands use of modern communications tools for sharing and collaborating with colleagues	
	• Exercises use of available technologies for broadcasting and disseminating information and knowledge	
Competency 8: To understand the ethical, legal, and sociopolitical aspects of information and its technologies	• Understands and respects concepts of information ownership	A,C
	• Recognizes one's rights and obligations under intellectual property and copyright laws	
	• Understands fair use and provides proper citations when referencing, sharing, or disseminating information	
	• Understands legal and ethical dimensions of plagiarism and how and why it should be avoided	
	• Appreciates implications underscoring information commodification and stratification of an information society	
Competency 9: To develop an appreciation of lifelong learning	• Perceives the importance of using information intelligently to remain knowledgeable in one's field	A,C
	• Recognizes need for and means of integrating accurate and timely information with technical and subject expertise	
	• Understands correlation between being information literate and taking a path of lifelong learning	

A = Theoretical/higher-level reasoning; B = Technical/psychomotor; C = Attitudinal/behavioral

- to organize and communicate information effectively;
- to appraise and evaluate the quality of information;
- to appreciate ethical, legal, and socioeconomic aspects of information and technologies; and
- to develop an appreciation for information literacy and lifelong learning.

By 2000, librarians had full responsibility for teaching HAS 363, *Computer Literacy for Healthcare Professionals,* a required, one-credit course. Developed in collaboration with clinical faculty, HAS 363 consisted of twenty-one credit hours of instruction through lectures and labs held over seven weeks. Students were grouped according to discipline. Specific learning objectives built cumulatively over the duration of the course. The course content for HAS 363 is summarized in Box 16.1.

EVALUATION METHODS

Direct participation in the education mission offers libraries opportunities to redefine their roles and reinvigorate their relevance to their parent institutions. However, faced with competition for access

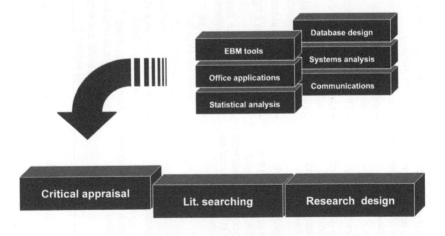

FIGURE 16.3. Module course development.

BOX 16.1. Outline of HAS 363

Week 1: Electronic information resources—searching PubMed, MEDLINE, CINAHL, and MD Consult, tracking citations in Web of Science, using the library's WebOPAC and electronic full-text books/journals.

Week 2: Evidence-based practice tools and strategies—searching ACP Journal Club Best Evidence, Cochrane Database of Systematic Reviews, and UpToDate, using the PICO model to form searchable clinical questions, examining strategies for appraising the validity and applicability of a research article to a clinical scenario.

Week 3: Professional presentation and communication—using PowerPoint, Publisher, Photo Editor, and Adobe Photoshop.

Week 4: Data management and statistical analysis—using Excel and SPSS statistics analysis software.

Week 5: Relational database theory and application, part 1—understanding table and query formation, data normalization, and relationship design.

Week 6: Relational database theory and application, part 2— using Access.

Week 7: Student research presentations

---

to the curricula, libraries must demonstrate measurably the efficacy of their instruction. Starting in 2000, outcomes-based evaluations were used at SBU to determine the degree to which course objectives were being achieved and to assess the effectiveness of library-based instruction. Three forms of data collection were used, including pre- and post-tests, student confidence inventories, and student course evaluations.

Pre- and Post-Tests

Pre- and post-tests gauged student acquisition of learned skills related to conducting literature searches. Pre-tests were administered prior to formal instruction. Post-tests were administered one week after the completion of the literature searching module. A second series of post-tests ("post5-test") was administered five weeks after the first post-test to measure skill retention. The pre-, post-, and post5-test instrument is featured in the Appendix. Data groups included the following:

- *Intervention group:* 179 usable pairings of pre-, post-, and post5-tests were gathered over a three-year period from 2000 to 2002 from 188 undergraduate OT, PT, and RT students.
- *Intervention subgroup:* thirty-three usable pairings of pre-, post-, and post5-tests were gathered in 2002 from approximately thirty-seven undergraduate OT and RT students.
- *Control group:* forty-eight usable pairings of pre-, post-, and post5-tests were gathered in 2002 from sixty-four undergraduate PA students.

The study design does not meet the criteria of a randomized controlled trial. Subjects were not randomized into study groups but were organized according to degree program. The study was single-blinded as identifiers, used to pair test results, were stripped before tests were scored. The intervention (instruction) group consisted of OT, PT, and RT students. A control group comprising PA students provided baseline comparison. For study purposes, PAs were comparable to OTs, PTs, and RTs, as all were undergraduates with similar program entrance requirements; all were enrolled simultaneously in the same prerequisite courses (e.g., anatomy, physiology, etc.); and until 2000, all were required to attend HAS 363. After 1999, scheduling restrictions forced the PA program administrators to withdraw their students from the course. Focal comparison is restricted to data gathered during the 2002 period, during which time pre- and post-tests were administered concurrently to the intervention subgroup and the control group. Table 16.2 shows subject distribution.

Scores shown are out of a possible 14. Pre-, post-, and post5-test results for the full intervention group are shown in Table 16.3. Results for the intervention subgroup and the control group are shown respectively in Table 16.3. Results for the full intervention group reveal appreciable variation in mean between the pre- ($M = 5.195$), post- ($M = .732$), and post5-tests ($M = 10.106$). Results for the intervention subgroup show even more significant change in mean: pre- ($M = 4.788$), post- ($M = 8.515$), and post5-tests ($M = 11.849$). Meanwhile, results in the control group do not show significant variation in mean between the pre- ($M = 3.271$), post- ($M = 3.854$), and post5-tests ($M = 3.375$).

TABLE 16.2. Distribution of usable test results by subjects.

	2000	2001	2002	Total
Intervention	75	71	33	179
Intervention subgroup	—	—	33	33
Control	0	0	48	48[a]

[a]Identifying a control group from among these students was not possible, due in part to scheduling difficulties and in part to the ethical dilemma of withholding instruction (the dependent variable) from a subgroup of students who would otherwise receive it.

TABLE 16.3. Group results.

	Mean	N	Std. deviation	Std. error mean
Intervention group (2000-2002) results				
Pre-test	5.195	179	3.110	.232
Post-test	9.732	179	7.514	.561
Post5-test	10.106	179	2.321	.232
Intervention subgroup (2002) results				
Pre-test	4.788	33	3.426	.596
Post-test	8.515	33	2.181	.378
Post5-test	11.849	33	2.451	.427
Control group (2002) results				
Pre-test	3.271	48	2.51582	.363
Post-test	3.854	48	2.90260	.419
Post5-test	3.375	48	2.87043	.414

As Table 16.4 reveals, paired t test analysis indicates that the mean score for the intervention group on the post-test ($M = 9.732$) was significantly greater at the $p < 0.01$ level (note: $t = 7.44$; $p < 0.001$) than the mean score on the pre-test ($M = 5.196$). The change is statistically significant and the null hypothesis can be rejected. As shown in Table 16.4, restricting analysis to the smaller intervention subgroup still allows rejection of the null hypothesis, since the mean post-test score ($M = 8.515$) was significantly greater at the $p < 0.01$ level (note: $t =$

TABLE 16.4. Group pairings.

| | Paired differences (99 percent confidence interval) | | | | | |
	Mean	Std. deviation	Std. error	*t*	Df	Sig (2-tailed)
Intervention group (2000-2002) pairings						
Pre-Post	4.536	8.161	.6099	7.437	178	<0.001
Pre-Post5	4.911	3.586	.2680	18.323	178	<0.001
Intervention subgroup (2002) pairings						
Pre-Post	3.727	3.430	.597	6.242	32	<0.001
Pre-Post5	7.060	3.766	.656	10.770	32	<0.001
Control group (2002) pairings						
Pre-Post	0.583	3.506	.506	1.153	47	0.255
Pre-Post5	0.104	4.421	.5827	0.163	47	0.871

6.242; $p < 0.001$) than the mean pre-test score ($M = 4.788$). The results demonstrate that instructional intervention by librarians had measurably effective results in student acquisition of searching skills. Moreover, analysis of pre- and post5-test pairings demonstrate student retention of acquired skills, given the elevated mean. Importantly, the narrowed standard deviation within the post5-test results reveal a greater central tendency toward the mean, thereby suggesting generalized improvement among the intervention groups. As shown in Table 16.4, results for the control group are not statistically significant.

These results suggest strongly the effectiveness of librarian intervention in both the acquisition and retention of learned skills. This contrasts with conclusions reached by Garg and Turtle, whose critical appraisal of earlier research found librarian instructional intervention to have only a moderate impact on initial literature skill acquisition and no impact on skill retention.[8] The observed variation may be attributable to the differences in the HSC Library courses and those courses studied by Garg and Turtle. In the former, literature searching was integrated into the larger course content and students acquired cumulative experiential understanding of its mechanics through the duration of the course. In the latter, literature searching alone was the main focus of the given class or workshop, lasting from one to eight hours. Students may be motivated to develop a better understanding of literature searching when instruction in this area is presented in a broader context, and when effective literature searches enable students to successfully complete other course requirements.

Pre- and Post-Course Confidence Inventories

Theorists have problematized a strictly quantifiable or "physicalist" approach to understanding information-seeking behavior.[9-10] Equally important is an understanding of the subject's sense of his or her own skill acquisition. For the study at hand, this was accomplished using a survey instrument to compare students' self-assessed confidence before and after the course. This pre- and post-course "confidence inventory" measured individual confidence according to various course parameters along an ordinal scale from 1 (very low to no confidence) to 4 (high confidence). Improvement in confidence was indicated in all areas of measure. Formal analysis of the pre- and post-course change in confidence (i.e., "I am able to conduct an effective search of biomedical and health care literature using bibliographic databases such as MEDLINE and CINAHL") yields a Pearson chi-square value of 11.07 (asymptotic significance = 0.001), suggesting a highly significant improvement in confidence. Table 16.5 provides a complete breakdown of the chi-square analysis of subjects' change in confidence for all seven parameters.

Student Evaluations

Using a five-point ordinal Likert scale ranging from "agree strongly" to "disagree strongly," students evaluated the course according to ten parameters shown in Table 16.6. Evaluations were positive. Students on average agreed or strongly agreed with all statements, affirming the recognized value and applicability of the course content and instruction.

Data gathered from these outcome measures demonstrated the success of the library-based education program and were used in part to argue persuasively for the expansion of the education mission of the HSC Library. In late 2000, a proposal was accepted to formalize the educational mission of the HSC Library by creating CHIE. Approval

TABLE 16.5. Chi-square analysis of confidence scales (N = 69).

	Pearson chi-square value	Asymp. sig (2-sided)	Contingency coefficient
I am able to recognize the importance of using clinical information/evidence-based recommendations in support of clinical decision making.	26.25	0.000	0.522
I am able to conduct an effective search of biomedical and healthcare literature using bibliographic databases such as MEDLINE and CINAHL.	11.07	0.001	0.370
I am able to recognize the relative strengths and limitations of evidence-based medicine review databases such as ACP Journal Club ("Best-Evidence") and Cochrane Database of Systematic Reviews as compared to MEDLINE.	12.20	0.016	0.385
I am able to differentiate between publication types such as a review article, a clinical trial, and a meta-analysis.	11.01	0.026	0.373
I am able to locate and evaluate high quality health care information on the Internet.[a]	1.149	0.563	0.563
I am able to organize and deliver a professional-quality presentation using MS PowerPoint.	14.64	0.002	0.416
I am able to organize clinical data using MS Excel (spreadsheet software) and/or MS Access (relational database software).	19.12	0.004	0.463

[a]Results demonstrate the instructional invention improved self-assessed confidence in subjects according to all areas of inquiry. The exception to this trend appears in the weak correlation in subject confidence locating and evaluating high-quality health care information on the Internet. The low Pearson value and the attributed asymptotic significance suggest that instruction had no appreciable influence in subject confidence. These results were, however, anticipated. The inclusion of this question in the survey offered a means of gauging instrument validity. For although the measure was retained on the survey instrument, the course content related to appraising Internet information resources was dropped from the course after 1999, to allow additional in-class coverage of other content. That the data do not support the conclusion that instruction improved confidence in the measured area is consistent with the fact that course instructional coverage was not provided in that area. Had the data suggested otherwise, the results from the rest of the instrument would have been thrown into question.

TABLE 16.6. Student evaluation (in percent).

	Agree strongly	Agree	Neutral	Disagree	Disagree strongly
Q1. Learning objectives for the program were clearly stated and addressed.	34	45	13	8	0
Q2. You have improved your skills and/or knowledge in the course's area of instruction.	40	43	7	7	3
Q3. Assignments were relevant to the course material and learning objectives.	20	58	12	14	6
Q4. Grading criteria for assignments and exercises were clearly communicated by instructor.	38	43	19	0	0
Q5. Assignments were graded fairly.	19	56	9	7	9
Q6. Instructor provided regular and timely feedback/grades on assignments and exercises.	12	65	14	0	9
Q7. Instructor was available and willing to provide assistance inside and outside of class.	33	38	27	2	0
Q8. Instructor communicated clearly.	56	37	7	0	0
Q9. Instructor demonstrated knowledge in the area of instruction.	72	18	8	2	0
Q10. Material taught in the course is relevant to your overall academic/ clinical training.	23	45	29	3	0

was received from the Office of the Vice President as well as from the respective deans of each of the HSC schools. Under the direction of a steering committee comprising representatives from each of the schools, CHIE was officially formed in fall 2001 with the following mandate:

- To integrate core informatics training into curricula of all HSC schools
- To host continuing education/continuing medical education (CE/CME) informatics training for practicing health professionals
- To assist HSC faculty to integrate technology in support of student learning

To secure the resources necessary to achieve CHIE's mission, the HSC Library first merged the formerly separate departments of Information Services and Education Services. CHIE was administered under a codirectorship, consisting of the former heads of the previously separate departments. Such organization helped invest all members of the new department with a sense of ownership of its mission and ameliorated staff anxiety about the merger. Priority for the new unit was given to development and delivery of curriculum integrated instruction, while traditional library public services (e.g., reference services) were scaled back significantly. For example, reference desk coverage was reduced from eighty-five to forty-nine hours per week over a three-year period.

To date, CHIE been successful in expanding deeper into the core curricula, especially in the schools of Health Technology and Management, Medicine, and Nursing, and to a lesser extent in Dental Medicine and Social Welfare. Schools are able to integrate informatics training without sustaining their own stand-alone informatics faculty and resources. Moreover, the central nature of CHIE is in keeping with the HSC's history of shared resources. Ultimately, it is anticipated that CHIE will become an informatics degree-granting arm of the HSC. At present, CHIE has become involved directly in providing required informatics training for new degree programs offered through the HSC, including new graduate programs such as the master's of public health (MPH) and doctorate of physical therapy (DPT). Current credit courses offered by CHIE members include:

Set #	Search History	Results
1	Breast neoplasms	3000
2	exp Breast neoplasms	3800
3	*Breast neoplasms	2400
4	*exp Breast neoplasms	3500
5	*exp Breast neoplasms/drug therapy	1600
6	*Tamoxifen	1100
7	*Tamoxifen/adverse effects	700
8	*exp Endometrial neoplasms	500
9	5 and 6	400
10	5 and 7 and 8	150

9. Set 2 contains more citations than Set 1. Why?
    A. ☐ Set 2 exploded breast neoplasms, retrieving subordinate concepts into the search
    B. ☐ Set 2 was entered after Set 1 and compiled additional materials to the first search
    C. ☐ Set 1 contains more relevant (or focused) articles than set 2
    D. ☐ Set 1 contains only peer-reviewed English-language articles on breast neoplasms
    E. ☐ I DO NOT KNOW

10. Set 3 contains fewer citations than Set 1. Why?
    A. ☐ Set 2 exploded breast neoplasms, retrieving subordinate concepts into the search
    B. ☐ Set 3 represents the articles in Set 2 not included in Set 2
    C. ☐ Set 3 contains more relevant (or focused) articles than Set 1
    D. ☐ Set 3 contains only peer-reviewed English-language articles on breast neoplasms
    E. ☐ I DO NOT KNOW

11. What is the nature of the citations retrieved in Set 5?
    A. ☐ Articles with a primary focus on drug therapy of all forms of breast neoplasms
    B. ☐ Articles with a primary focus on drug therapy of breast neoplasms in women
    C. ☐ Articles from dealing with Phase IV clinical trials of breast cancer drugs
    D. ☐ Articles with a primary focus on diet therapy of all forms of breast neoplasms
    E. ☐ I DO NOT KNOW

12. What is the nature of the citations retrieved in Set 10?
    A. ☐ Articles dealing with drug therapy of breast neoplasms or endometrial neoplasms
    B. ☐ Articles about therapy of breast neoplasms
    C. ☐ Articles relating tamoxifen therapy for breast cancer with endometrial cancer
    D. ☐ Articles addressing dosing regimes for administration of tamoxifen
    E. ☐ I DO NOT KNOW

13. Shade in the appropriate area of the **Venn diagram** below so as to represent the search results from Set 10.

Set 5
*exp breast neoplasms /drug therapy

Set 7
*Tamoxifen /adverse effect

Set 8
*exp endometrial neoplasms

☐ I DO NOT KNOW

14. In THEORY, what is the LARGEST POSSIBLE number of citations that COULD be retrieved from combining Set 1 with Set 7 using the Boolean logical operator **AND** (i.e , entering the command **1 AND 7**)?
    A. ☐ 3000
    B. ☐ 3700
    C. ☐ 2300
    D. ☐ 700
    E. ☐ I DO NOT KNOW

NOTES

1. Elder, Owen C. and Nick, Todd. "Moving Toward a Core Curriculum in Schools of the Allied Health Professions: Knowledge and Skills Considered Important by Department Chairs in Four Disciplines." *Journal of Allied Health* 26(Spring 1997):51-56.

2. American Occupational Therapy Association. *Standards for an Accredited Educational Program for the Occupational Therapist*. Bethesda, MD: American Occupational Therapy Association, 1997.

3. American Physical Therapy Association. *Evaluative Criteria for Accreditation of Education Programs for the Preparation of Physical Therapists*. Alexandria, VA: American Physical Therapy Association, 1998.

4. National Board for Respiratory Care. *Credentialing for the Respiratory Care Profession*. Lenexa, KS: National Board for Respiratory Care, 2003.

5. Association of Health Sciences Libraries. *Annual Statistics of Medical School Libraries in the United States and Canada, 2000-01*. Twenty-Fourth Edition. Seattle, WA: Association of Academic Health Sciences Libraries, 2001.

6. Association of Health Sciences Libraries. *Annual Statistics of Medical School Libraries in the United States and Canada, 1995-96*. Eighteenth Edition. Seattle, WA: Association of Academic Health Sciences Libraries, 1996.

7. Gibson, Kenneth E.; and Silverberg, Michael. "A Two-Year Experience Teaching Computer Literacy to First-Year Medical Students Using Skills-Based Cohorts." *Bulletin of the Medical Library Association* 88(April 2000):157-164.

8. Garg, J. and Turtle, K.M. "Effective of Training Health Professionals in Literature Search Skills Using Electronic Health Databases: A Critical Appraisal." *Health Information and Libraries Journal* 20(2003):33-41.

9. Budd, J. "Information Seeking in Theory and Practice: Rethinking Public Services in Libraries." *Reference and User Services Quarterly* 40(2001):256-263.

10. Ellis, D. "Modeling the Information Seeking Patterns of Academic Researchers: A Grounded Theory Approach." *Library Quarterly* 63(1993):469-486.

Chapter 17

Integrating Medical Informatics into the School of Medicine Curriculum at the University of California, San Francisco

Keir Reavie
Gail L. Persily
Kevin H. Souza

INTRODUCTION

In September 2001, the University of California, San Francisco (UCSF), School of Medicine (SOM) implemented Essential Core, a new preclinical curriculum for incoming medical students. Simultaneously, the school redesigned its clinical core curriculum for third-year students and enhanced the fourth year by adding "advanced studies" tracks based on disciplines such as humanities and medicine, and global and public health.

Essential Core is designed to provide a more interdisciplinary approach to medical education by fully integrating basic, social, behavioral, and clinical sciences and introducing students to the patient care environment from the beginning of their medical education.[1-2] Essential Core also reduces didactic lectures in favor of more self-directed, small-group, and hands-on learning. Much of the self-directed and hands-on learning is facilitated through the use of clinical case studies, which the students work on throughout the curriculum. Cases are carefully designed to teach students basic and clinical sciences knowledge required to answer clinical questions presented by the cases.

Students participate in problem-based learning (PBL) sessions throughout the first two years of the curriculum. The PBL sessions also use clinical cases, from which students develop their own questions and learning opportunities through discussion among themselves and with the facilitator of the small group. Students then use these questions to conduct their own self-directed learning in basic and clinical sciences. The use of clinical cases in the curriculum engages students in solving clinical problems on a regular basis, preparing them for third- and fourth-year clinical studies. As part of this learning process, faculty involved in designing the new curriculum recognized that student success in dealing with problems presented by clinical cases depends on their skills in accessing, retrieving, managing, using, and communicating information. Within this environment, medical informatics plays an important role early in medical education.

Along with the new curriculum, in September 2001 the SOM introduced an electronic curriculum (iROCKET) using an online learning management system. iROCKET facilitates student ability to engage in self-directed learning outside the regular lectures, labs, and small-group sessions (Figure 17.1). It also assists in the integration of informatics into the curriculum, since little didactic time is available, and small-group sessions are difficult to schedule due to limited numbers of librarians and computer-based classrooms. Dividing the entire first-year class of 141 students into groups of twenty and conducting hands-on computer labs requires three to five simultaneous sessions with two instructors assigned to each.

Using the clinical cases and iROCKET with a combination of lectures, demonstrations, and hands-on computer labs, librarians and faculty at UCSF worked collaboratively to develop a medical informatics syllabus that is integrated across the curriculum, rather than developing an individual course or series of courses on informatics. Creating a longitudinal theme for informatics in a medical school curriculum is not unique. The recent trend of medical schools to modify their traditional didactic curriculum with other teaching methods has created an environment where integration can easily take place.[3-4] Curriculum integration, particularly by attaching informatics learning opportunities to clinical case studies, creates the relevant background for this topic, and an environment in which the students better

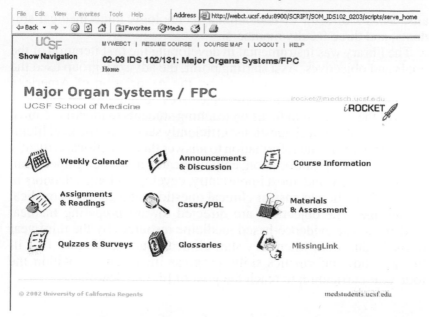

FIGURE 17.1. iROCKET—Major Organ Systems Web page.

understand why they are learning to retrieve, analyze, and use information.

This chapter discusses the participation of UCSF librarians in the development of the medical informatics curriculum. Specifics include the development of goals and learning objectives; creation of syllabi; delivery of informatics content via iROCKET; lessons learned from integrating informatics into the new curriculum; and plans for modifying the future curriculum.

EDUCATIONAL APPROACHES

Developing Goals and Objectives

Development of the new curriculum began several years before implementation in September 2001. The first step was for the multidisciplinary advisory group appointed by the SOM to develop goals and learning objectives. The advisory group consisted of two librarians, SOM's director of educational technology, three medical students, and three faculty members.

The library was instrumental in developing the first iteration of the goals and objectives. As a starting point, the advisory group used the information objectives developed by the Association of American Medical Colleges.[5] The learning objectives outlined for the first two years of the curriculum focus on teaching students to identify clinical problems; ask clinical questions; efficiently search the medical literature; retrieve relevant information to answer their questions; critically evaluate retrieved information; communicate knowledge gained from the information; and, most importantly, develop lifelong behaviors in using information to answer clinical questions and gain new medical knowledge. The objectives are directed toward preparing medical students to use evidence-based medicine resources by the third year of their education, when they start clinical rotations. Figure 17.2 illustrates how informatics skills progress incrementally within the four-year curriculum to reach the goal of lifelong learning.

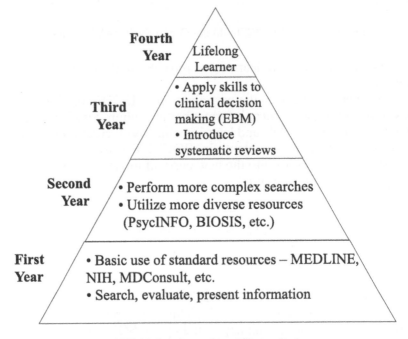

FIGURE 17.2. Informatics skills curriculum.

The advisory group discussed the first iteration of the goals and learning objectives during several meetings and via e-mail. Finalized goals and learning objectives were presented to a cross-section of faculty and students involved in designing the new curriculum. Course committees consisting of faculty and students met regularly to develop various portions of the curriculum for the first year. Members of several different advisory groups met with these committees to discuss the integration of various topics across the curriculum. Examples of integrated topics include medical informatics, behavioral and social sciences, and bioethics. Once the goals and objectives for the medical informatics component of the curriculum were widely disseminated and discussed, librarians in the advisory group began working with smaller groups of faculty and students responsible for designing specific teaching sessions in order to integrate portions of the informatics syllabus. In developing the syllabus, the advisory group focused on specific objectives outlined in the advisory group document, to ensure all objectives would be addressed in the first two years of the curriculum.

Following the first-year experiences integrating informatics into the curriculum, and through further discussion with faculty and students, the learning objectives were revised (see Appendix A). The medical informatics advisory group realized early on that the first version of the goals and objectives was very ambitious. The current iteration of the goals and learning objectives is more realistic, although still somewhat ambitious, about the way medical students work and what they are expected to learn in the first two years of medical school. The goals and objectives are a work in progress that will be revised again as informatics is integrated into the full four years of the medical school curriculum.

Integrating into the Curriculum

As mentioned previously, various methods have been used to integrate the informatics syllabus throughout the curriculum, including lectures and demonstrations, hands-on computer workshops, self-directed learning using iROCKET, and informatics assignments associated with clinical cases. Each informatics component builds on previous syllabi. Over time, the syllabus becomes more sophisticated in its use of information resources, student assignments, and how students critically evaluate and use information. As the syllabus progresses through the curriculum, it also contains fewer lectures, demonstrations, and hands-on computer workshops. Learning becomes increasingly self-directed. As student informatics skills improve, instructors depend on iROCKET to provide just-in-time assistance and feedback to students. Throughout this process, the focus is on meeting the goals objectives outlined for the curriculum, even as those goals and objectives are modified.

Since the new curriculum launched in fall 2001, informatics learning objectives have been incorporated into seven teaching sessions with a total of eight hours of didactic and hands-on instruction.[6] The following four examples describe modules integrated into the first year of Essential Core.

Example 1: Medical Informatics Orientation

In September 2001, the first-year medical students received an introduction to the medical literature and key resources for accessing the literature, within a small-group computer workshop. To reach all 141 medical students, two computer labs accommodating 18 students each were used simultaneously during four two-hour periods, with workshops stretching over two days. Sessions were conducted with a minimum of four instructors, with two scheduled for each lab.

Instructors (in this case, librarians) for these sessions discussed the life cycle of medical literature from the first reports of clinical research in journal articles to standard medical knowledge in textbooks and other basic medical reference materials. Students were introduced to the library catalog, online medical textbooks such as the MD Consult collection, and key reference sources (*5 Minute Clinical Consult,* PubMed MEDLINE, etc.). This session was a combination lecture and demonstration on accessing and searching the resources. Since the sessions were held in computer labs, students also had time to search resources on their own and ask questions. The students then completed an assignment consisting of questions derived from the first clinical case used in the curriculum. The case is an emergency medicine event (a motorcycle accident victim) that facilitates learning in anatomy, physiology, and clinical assessment. Assignment questions were designed to introduce students to the basics such as locating books in the library, using an online textbook, and performing a basic MEDLINE search. The goal of this exercise was to help students distinguish among different literature resources and the different types of medical information contained in each. Completed assignments were sent by e-mail to instructors, who reviewed them and provided feedback to the entire class.

Materials for this session were also available on iROCKET, enabling students to review the class contents and get help with the assignment. iROCKET included instructions and direct links to resources needed to complete the assignment. Students could also use iROCKET to communicate electronically with instructors, if needed. Once instructors reviewed the completed assignments, feedback was posted in iROCKET's online discussion forums, which was easily accessible to the students.

Example 2: Introduction to Problem-Based Learning

Based on the experience of integrating informatics into the curriculum for the first time, librarians worked with faculty to change the introductory medical informatics session for the first-year medical students in September 2002. The most obvious basis for the success of informatics in a medical school curriculum was making it relevant for the students. The introductory session needed to be more closely tied to PBL, which requires students to continually use information resources for self-directed learning.

Librarians worked closely with faculty to coordinate a combination of PBL small-group sessions and hands-on computer workshops, introduce students to the concept of PBL, and discuss resources to research learning issues generated by PBL cases throughout the Essential Core. To link the computer labs to the small-group sessions, four simultaneous computer labs with a minimum of eight instructors (two for each lab) were held. Since eight librarians were not available for these sessions, faculty and librarians teamed up to conduct the computer labs.

Students attended a brief lecture that described the PBL process and how it worked. The students then broke into smaller discussion groups to talk about a case and identify relevant learning issues. The main goal of the session was to make the students familiar with the process. The students took the learning issues and questions to the computer labs. Librarian instructors introduced students to key resources (online medical reference tools and textbooks, MEDLINE) to be used to answer these questions. The students used time in the lab to work on these questions or asked the instructors questions about using the resources. This lab time was also used to give students some hands-on experience using iROCKET. They were required to post at least one learning issue to the iROCKET discussion forum.

Example 3: Locating Clinical Research

Approximately two months after the introductory informatics workshop, students completed their second informatics session. This session was closely tied to a clinical case being used in the curriculum. At this time, students learned about the major organ systems. The case involved a cardiovascular patient. Students attended a combination lecture and demonstration on searching MEDLINE. They also completed an assignment in which they were guided to ask specific clinical questions presented by the case, which they tried to answer by searching online textbooks and MEDLINE. Because the patient in this case had hypertension, the questions revolved around drug therapy for hypertension and the prevention of future coronary events. Appendix B features the informatics assignment for major organ systems. Objectives of this session were to increase sophistication using online textbooks and the PubMed search interface, including using Medical Subject Headings (MeSH) and limits to help narrow searches and retrieve articles reporting clinically relevant information.

The assignments for this session were completed before students attend small-group sessions to discuss the clinical case in more detail. Students were expected to use this as a learning opportunity, not only to search for answers to these clinical questions, but to use the information found to facilitate discussion during small-group sessions.

Again, iROCKET provided students with help and instructions for completing the assignment, as well as feedback after assignments have been reviewed by instructors. The first time this session was offered, the students worked on a collection of questions. The time spent by a single librarian reviewing these assignments and preparing the feedback was substantial, requiring almost two weeks. When the session was offered again in 2002, students worked in groups (two to four students) on one of four questions related to the case. Four librarians each reviewed a single question and compiled the feedback. This helped streamline the review and feedback process considerably.

Example 4: Using Key Internet Resources

The third informatics session was a hands-on computer workshop linked with a clinical case involving a cancer patient. Workshop instructors were both librarians and faculty from the department of epidemiology. The objectives of this session were to introduce students to the primary information resources for access to cancer and related information, including cancer.gov, the Centers for Disease Control, and PubMed, and to review criteria for evaluating the accuracy and reliability of resources on the Internet.

Logistically, the small-group hands-on workshops were coordinated as in the first example, but in this case, rather than a lecture and demonstration of resources, students used the two-hour lab to work through a series of questions related to the cancer case, including epidemiological questions on cancer prevalence and mortality. Students used a variety of resources to answer the questions, and thus gained familiarity with valuable tools to be used in a future cancer PBL case. Librarians and faculty worked together on each session to answer student questions about the assignment and resources being used to complete it. iROCKET provided access to the assignment, hints for its completion, and links to relevant resources. Students were required to hand in a completed assignment at the end of the workshop. These were reviewed by faculty and librarians, but in this instance, no feedback was provided to students.

DISCUSSION

The first challenge that UCSF librarians faced integrating medical informatics across the curriculum was the difficulty of working with the large numbers of faculty and students involved in this process. Each course had two course directors and approximately 100 faculty involved in teaching the course. Course committees developed large thematic portions of the curriculum that integrate numerous disciplines. Collaborating with a group of faculty and students was very different from working with a single course director, whose attention may be easier to obtain.

An important aspect of meeting with committees and gaining attention for informatics was to get support from the faculty and administrators responsible for overseeing the development of the entire curriculum. This encouraged the curriculum committees to include informatics in their planning. On the plus side, working with large committees made integration easier, since it was more likely that some committee members understood the importance of medical informatics in the curriculum.

iROCKET helped to integrate informatics into a curriculum that overall had far less didactic time and more self-directed learning. iROCKET was also useful in allowing a small number of librarian instructors to interact with numerous students. iROCKET helps instructors provide assignments tied to cases, enables students to obtain help with the assignments, and assists with communication between students and instructors. Students can submit assignments, and obtain feedback from instructors. In addition, iROCKET enables librarians to post course content directly, which makes for an efficient process when collaborating with many faculty.

Librarians and faculty quickly learned that medical informatics must be associated closely to clinical cases in the curriculum, so that students see the relevance of informatics skills and do not view the assignments as busy work. In particular, students realized that PBL offered excellent opportunities to reinforce informatics skills within the context of coursework that required them to search the literature, evaluate its relevance, present information in a cohesive manner, and cite sources. This realization precipitated the development of a PBL orientation, providing important context for student introduction to library resources and related tools.

Initially, feedback for the assignments was slow because of the time required to review all assignments and write the feedback with limited library personnel. Informatics assignments were rethought and removed completely from the informatics orientation, which then focused on using resources for PBL.

In "Example 3: Locating Clinically Applicable Information," changes were also made. Rather than working on a series of questions related to a case, groups of students now work on a single question. With fewer assignments to review, librarians review individual questions from approximately 25 percent of the class, spreading this work more thinly.

The assignment feedback discussed common problems identified in the assignments, including asking overly complex questions; improperly using MeSH; "inventing" MeSH terms to perform a search, rather than looking them up; and performing far too broad a subject search to identify relevant articles. The feedback also provided examples of well-phrased questions and appropriate search strategies to answer them.

In reviewing the citations in the assignments, librarians realized that first-year medical students are more focused on using standard medical information resources such as medical textbooks than more sophisticated research resources such as MEDLINE. This was confirmed through ongoing discussion with faculty and students. During the first two years of medical education, students are directed more toward textbooks than MEDLINE. Although students should be knowledgeable about searching MEDLINE by the time they enter clinical rotations in the third year, they do not view this as a priority until rotations start. In the third year of medical school at UCSF, students receive more in-depth education on evidence-based medicine and making clinical decisions. At that time, sophisticated MEDLINE search skills are needed to efficiently locate clinical research. This finding in particular led the advisory group to rewrite the medical informatics goals and learning objectives for the first two years of the curriculum.

CONCLUSION

The multidisciplinary group represented faculty, students, and librarians interested in developing a medical informatics curriculum. The AAMC document on medical informatics objectives[5] helped the advisory group develop informatics goals and learning objectives for the new medical school curriculum at UCSF. Informatics knowledge and skills increased gradually over time, as students became more efficient in accessing, retrieving, managing, and evaluating information related to patient care. Because the process is ongoing, clinical cases and iROCKET can be used to facilitate self-directed and lifelong learning processes.

The next step is to develop syllabi for third- and fourth-year programs. In addition, formal measurement of student informatics abilities needs to take place, as well as objective evaluation of the current medical informatics curriculum. At the end of the second year, students have an option to test their search skills using a self-evaluation test on iROCKET. This evaluation will be formalized so that skills can be reviewed and graded by instructors, not unlike taking an exam. Evaluation will be important to help modify and expand medical informatics in the curriculum over the next several years.

APPENDIX A: OBJECTIVES FOR A MEDICAL INFORMATICS COMPONENT IN THE ESSENTIAL CORE CURRICULUM

Medical Informatics Advisory Group
School of Medicine, University of California, San Francisco

The educational goal for the medical informatics component in the Essential Core Curriculum is to prepare medical school graduates to be lifelong learners who use information efficiently to make patient care decisions. Students must have the skills to retrieve and assess reliable information. By the end of the second year of medical school, students should be prepared to use these skills and to then apply knowledge acquired from reliable information resources in medical practice.

Year I

The goals for Year I of the Essential Core Curriculum are to familiarize medical students with the key resources for access to reliable medical and health sciences information; to provide them with an understanding of how to select the appropriate information resources to answer different kinds of questions; and to develop their skills using technology to access, retrieve, and manage information for their work.

Objectives for Year I

At the end of Year I, medical students should be able to do the following:

- Explain the publication, dissemination, and knowledge cycle of health sciences information
- Explain the types of information resources that are available (books, journals, secondary resources such as the MEDLINE database, etc.) and the kinds of information that can be found in each
- Identify the correct resource to retrieve relevant information to solve specific health care questions
- Formulate search strategies to retrieve relevant published medical literature
- Locate books and other materials in the library
- Quickly access relevant information in medical textbooks
- Run a literature search on the MEDLINE database
- Access key Web sites to locate high-quality health information for clinical professionals and patients
- Evaluate Web sites for dependability in the information they provide

- Identify and use bibliographic databases other than MEDLINE to obtain health sciences information
- Consolidate a variety of information from diverse resources and clearly present this information to their colleagues

Year II

The goal of the medical informatics curriculum in Year II is to enable medical students to efficiently retrieve reliable clinical research from a variety of resources. By the end of the second year, students will be proficient in accessing reliable evidence and will be prepared to analyze the evidence and acquire knowledge that can then be applied to clinical decision making.

Objectives for Year II

At the end of Year II, medical students should be able to do the following:

- Identify high-quality resources that present evidence on the effects of clinical interventions
- Ask a clinical question that can be answered by the health science literature
- Efficiently retrieve the best clinical evidence at the point of patient care
- Search MEDLINE and other high-quality clinical information resources to retrieve information that can be applied in clinical practice
- Effectively use advanced computer software tools (e.g., spreadsheet, database management, and bibliographic management software) to manage and manipulate data and information
- Manipulate data and information to acquire knowledge and support hypotheses regarding patient care
- Communicate data, information, and other findings derived from their research in oral and written formats to help educate others

APPENDIX B: *MAJOR ORGAN SYSTEMS MEDICAL INFORMATICS ASSIGNMENT*

DUE DATE: Monday, November 25, 2002, 10 a.m.

GRADE: Complete or Incomplete

Please read the entire assignment carefully before starting.

The purpose of this assignment is to help develop your skills in searching for medical information to support clinical interventions and reporting what you learned from the information retrieved. Completing this assignment will help prepare you to discuss the Mr. Jackson case in your small groups on Monday and Tuesday.

Work on this assignment in groups of two to four students. Your group should consist of people from your assigned small group. Select only one of the following questions to research. It should not take you much more than an hour to complete the research and write a brief report on your findings.

Questions

Mr. Jackson has received or is receiving the following medical interventions.

1. Percutaneous transluminal coronary angioplasty to treat unstable angina.
2. Atenolol to control hypertension.
3. Simvastatin to control hyperlipidemia.
4. Aspirin to prevent angina.

Each group of students should select one intervention of interest. Research the evidence to support the intervention being used for Mr. Jackson's conditions.

Instructions

Each group will hand in a brief report of their research. Include a *statement of the clinical question you are trying to answer,* and the names of all students that worked on the report. E-mail the report to <keir.reavie@ library.ucsf.edu>.

The report should be in the following format:

1. A brief discussion of the evidence that supports the intervention you have researched.
2. A list of citations for your sources of information. For each citation, include a brief note on which resource you used to locate the source cited, and how you found the source (i.e., I located the source in MD Consult using the search term *hypertension,* or I located in the source

in MEDLINE using the MeSH search term *hypertension*). When citing your sources, use the guidelines outlined in the *Use of References* document.

The reports will be reviewed and feedback will be provided to the class via the Library Assignment discussion group on iROCKET.

Helpful Hints

If you are unfamiliar with some of the terms in the research questions or need background information on a drug or surgical procedure, use the medical encyclopedia available on MedlinePlus. If you use MedlinePlus, indicate that you have used it to obtain background information and note the topic you researched.

Use Harrison's Online and MD Consult to obtain standard drug information (indications, administration, and dosage), practice guidelines, and treatment overviews.

Using an electronic resource is not always the best and/or easiest way to find answers to clinical questions. You can also use the UCSF Library Catalog to locate information in print formats within the library.

For more in-depth and current research on these interventions and their outcomes, search the journal literature referenced in the MEDLINE database using PubMed@UCSF.

Resources for This Assignment

- Introduction to Formulating a Clinical Question
- MedlinePlus
- UCSF Library Catalog
- Textbooks:
    Harrison's Principles of Internal Medicine
    MD Consult (contains a variety of textbooks and drug information)
- The journal literature:
    MEDLINE on PubMed@UCSF
    PubMed@UCSF Quick Guide
    Detailed guide to searching MEDLINE
- *Use of References*

Additional Help

If you require additional help or have any questions about this assignment, please use the Library Assignment discussion list available in the Announcements and Discussion section of iROCKET. An instructor will respond to your questions as soon as possible.

NOTES

1. Irby, D.M. and Wilkerson, L. "Educational Innovations in Academic Medicine and Environmental Trends." *Journal of General Internal Medicine* 18(2003):370-376.

2. Hollander, H., Loeser, H., and Irby, D. "An Anticipatory Quality Improvement Process for Curricular Reform." *Academic Medicine* 77(2002):930.

3. Edward G. Miner Library, University of Rochester Medical Center. *Informatics Competencies for Medical Students at the University of Rochester Medical Center: Planning Document, 1995.* Available: <http://www.urmc.rochester.edu/Miner/Educ/medinfostudents1.html>.

4. Burrows, S., Moore, K., Arriaga, J., Paulaitis, G., and Lemkau, H.L. "Developing an 'Evidence-Based Medicine and Use of the Biomedical Literature' Component As a Longitudinal Theme of an Outcomes-Based Medical School Curriculum: Year 1." *Journal of the Medical Library Association* 91(January 2003):34-41.

5. Association of American Medical Colleges. *Contemporary Issues in Medicine: Medical Informatics and Population Health.* Washington, DC: Association of American Medical Colleges, 1998. Available: <http://www.aamc.org/meded/msop/msop2.pdf>.

6. School of Medicine, University of California, San Francisco. *Ilios: UCSF School of Medicine Curriculum Management Tool.* San Francisco, CA: School of Medicine, University of California, San Francisco, 2002. Available: <http://medschool.ucsf.edu/ilios/>.

Chapter 18

ThinkPads, Medical Education, and the Library at Wake Forest University

David C. Stewart

INTRODUCTION

In 1996, the Committee on Educational Computing Recommendations of the Wake Forest University School of Medicine (WFUSM) specified information management goals for the School of Medicine curriculum, including basic information literacy, basic computer literacy, computer-aided learning and evaluation, communication, information retrieval and management, and patient management.

When the undergraduate campus of Wake Forest University implemented its plan to give a computer to each freshman, the medical school decided to integrate portable computing into the medical curriculum as a way of achieving its information management goals. The Mobile Computing Project (also known as the ThinkPad Project) first met in January 1997. Comprising representatives from IBM, Office of Medical Education, Information Services, Biomedical Communications, Physician Assistant Program, and Coy C. Carpenter Library, the project's immediate objective was to provide laptop computers, along with the necessary training, to the incoming members of the physician assistant (PA) class of 1998. The PA program was chosen as the pilot project because of the small number of students, its location in a building separate from the medical school, and the commitment of its faculty to the implementation of a computer-based curriculum. The library was chosen, in part, because of its past educational programs and projects, which included computer training in a funded pilot program with the Department of Family and Community

Medicine for WFUSM problem-based-learning curriculum medical students in 1994.

EDUCATIONAL APPROACHES

At the time the Mobile Computing Project began, there was no network, no support staff, and no one agency responsible for training faculty, staff, and students in this new technology. By the end of the first year, the task force had created an academic network, identified support staff, and given the library the responsibility for computer training of the incoming students.

The training work group's first task was to identify the groups in need of training, which products would require instruction, and how and when that training would be delivered. Faculty and students were two obvious groups to teach. It was easy to assess the PA faculty's needs since there were only six instructors and face-to-face meetings could be arranged quickly and easily. Training in computer basics such as Windows operations and e-mail applications was quickly identified. A key training need was the conversion of class syllabi to the Lotus Notes–based template adopted by the undergraduate campus the year before. The WFU template organized classroom materials such as course syllabi and bibliographies into "cabinets" only accessible to members of that course. E-mail and calendar functions were part of the template as well. Class members could read materials, correspond with each other, and work collaboratively.

Early in April 1997, PA faculty and staff took part in training sessions that covered several areas: communications (e-mail, Word), computer literacy (Windows 95, Lotus Notes), curriculum (WFU template), information retrieval (MEDLINE, Reference Manager), and instructional aids (Excel, PowerPoint). Librarians, CyberSkills staff (a local computer-training company contracted to provide application software instruction for the Medical Center), and Biomedical Communications staff were enlisted to provide this training.

Students were expected to have a wider range of needs than faculty. So that the trainers could prepare, a survey was included in the pre-enrollment packet traditionally mailed to the new PA students twelve weeks before orientation. The incoming forty-eight students were asked about the following skills and knowledge:

- Ability to perform basic computer operations
- Ability to perform various word processing operations
- Ability to use Lotus Notes
- Types of training that would be beneficial
- Word processing applications used
- Ways in which computers were used
- Expectations and concerns about the ThinkPad Project

Survey Results

The forty-seven surveys returned indicated a wide range of abilities. Almost all students could turn on a computer, use a mouse, use a diskette, launch applications, and perform basic file maintenance activities, but few could perform advanced file maintenance activities or use e-mail, Web browsers, or electronic databases. All but four of the incoming students reported having good word processing skills, while forty-seven reported little or no knowledge of Lotus Notes. When the students were asked to indicate how training should be delivered, no one training type (organized classes, written materials from the school, online tutorials, or software manuals) stood out as a clear favorite. Even when organized classes received a noticeable majority of responses (Lotus Notes and electronic databases), numerous respondents also marked the other training types.

Student replies to questions about expectations and concerns indicated that they expected computer technology to add a great deal to their education by increasing access to information, enhancing communication among classmates and instructors, and reducing the number of books they would have to buy. Concerns centered on the fear that their computer skills would be inadequate to deal with the demands of the program. The responses indicated a need to give students enough applicability to convince them of the technology's usefulness, and that training needed to be thorough and effective in order to allay students' fears that they lacked the necessary computer skills to succeed in their coursework.

The training group felt that it was most important that all students be at or near the same level of computer proficiency at the end of the orientation period. Proficiency was defined as familiarity with unique IBM laptop features such as the Track Point, and also the ability to open, move, and copy files and folders; to back up files; and to enter, maneuver, open attachments, and communicate in the WFU template. Since the template was created as a Lotus Notes application, separate sessions were scheduled for Lotus Notes instruction.

An evaluation form was created to assess the effectiveness of the training. Levels of proficiency needed to be assessed at the end of orientation, so a survey, similar to the one the students had answered in the pre-enrollment package, was scheduled for a later time within the first semester. Sessions were scheduled for the distribution of the laptops and for teaching Windows, file management, and Lotus Notes. Other sessions dealing with specific software applications such as Word and PowerPoint would be scheduled later in the fall.

IBM personnel conducted the computer distribution on the first day of orientation week. The students were divided into two groups, with one group meeting at 1:00 p.m. and the other at 3:00 p.m., to receive their computers and instructions in the proper care and handling of them. The next morning, the students were taught Windows/File Management. The class was split into two halves. The first half (twenty-four students) arrived at 8:00 a.m. and were immediately divided into four groups of six. Each of these four groups met with a librarian in a separate small-group room. At the end of these sessions, everyone regrouped in the large PA classroom, with the trainers conducting twelve exercises based upon this material (see Appendix A). This whole process was then repeated with the second half of the class at 10:00 a.m. The Lotus Notes sessions were scheduled over the next three afternoons. One-third of the class at a time attended a two-hour session that covered the basics of Lotus Notes, including its e-mail and calendar functions and how the WFU template worked. The week's training sessions were evaluated using a printed form consisting of seven questions; five of the questions were multiple choice and the other two questions were short answer (see Appendix B).

New Medical Curriculum

In 1998, the second year of the project, library staff planned not only PA student orientation week but the medical student orientation week as well. In 1998, medical students were introduced to a new curriculum as well as new technology.

The new medical curriculum incorporated a small-group structure in the first two years of study. Groups of six medical students met on

.Mondays with two faculty tutors and were given a case. During the week, students identified learning issues and returned on Friday to discuss those learning issues. The library training group decided to incorporate the small-group concept into the medical student's orientation.

In the previous year, the distribution of computers to PA students was handled by the IBM staff in two sessions of twenty-four students each. A distinct disadvantage of this approach was that the number of students in a session was too large for the IBM staff to handle the number of questions asked. Also, as an individual question was answered, the group's focus shifted away from the instructor and the training issues, making it more difficult, each time a new question was raised, to stay on topic.

The incoming medical student class size was 108, more than twice the size of the PA class. The medical students were asked to meet in their small-group rooms with their fellow group members, with no more than six members in a group. They learned how to connect to the network, how to connect laptops to the video monitor, and how to connect to Softboard (an interactive display board found in each small-group room). More personalized instruction related to using the laptop and its functions was offered. The Windows training and exercises of the previous year were folded into this session, which lasted ninety minutes.

The training script outlined all desired content for the laptop distribution session, as every student needed to come away with the same basic information, covered in the same way. In training the librarian trainers, it was helpful to refer to the ThinkPad Technology Guide, written by the undergraduate campus staff. Many students had no familiarity with laptop computers, much less the IBM version of one. A written script, outlining every step within the distribution session, would ensure that all essential points would be covered as well as giving the trainer examples to follow when demonstrating a special feature of the laptop or a program such as *Stedman's Medical Dictionary*. The annotated script became one of the constants in the computer training from year to year.

The medical students also attended two two-hour sessions later in the week. These large-group sessions focused on materials that did not need as much individual instruction and covered fewer topics than the small-group sessions. One session was devoted to Lotus Notes, the other session to Netscape e-mail, Web browsing, and MEDLINE searching. Each of these sessions had roughly one-quarter of the total freshman class (twenty-seven students). The new PA students followed the same format two weeks later. Again, evaluations were conducted using a printed form with the same questions as the previous year. The initial faculty training sessions occurred in May, since many faculty members would not be available during the summer. This training consisted of an introduction to the laptop's features and the unique software programs loaded on it, plus a discussion of how the emerging academic network would work during the semester. During orientation week, additional faculty training sessions were held that covered the specific instructional technologies available in the small-group rooms.

Student Trainers

The third year's training in 1999 followed the same format with one new twist; second-year medical students served as trainers for the basic computer distribution class. Advantages included second-year students' familiarity with the laptops, small-group rooms, and the first-year course of study. New students were most enthusiastic about the student trainers, and this practice has been continued every year since. The student trainers are given the script and expected to cover all of its points, while also sharing some of their first-year experiences with the new students. The training work group continues to train the trainers in an effort to provide consistent instruction from year to year.

In year four of the project, the university abandoned the Lotus Notes–based WFU template, altering the focus of the large-group sessions. Because the WFU template incorporated a scheduling feature, its retirement necessitated teaching the Netscape calendar. Over the previous year, the newly formed Academic Computing department had created a Web-based curriculum shell that held course information and adjunct materials much like the discarded WFU template. Academic Computing staff demonstrated this new tool to the students. Librarians already teaching Netscape e-mail and calendar functions in regularly scheduled classes to the Medical Center's staff were assigned to teach this material to the students. Since the new curriculum template demanded a considerable amount of time to demonstrate, the calendaring segment was incorporated into the Netscape e-mail, Web browsing, and MEDLINE session.

This arrangement was modified in year five when Netscape e-mail and calendar were shifted to the Web curriculum session. The time saved in the MEDLINE session allowed the trainers to introduce the students to the growing number of Web resources purchased by the library, including electronic textbooks and journals, which also fit more appropriately into the MEDLINE session. A simulated case was given to the students after the MEDLINE and electronic textbooks demonstration. Groups of four or five students collaborated in finding the answers to a series of questions based upon the case. Students were encouraged to look for the answers in the electronic textbooks by searching MEDLINE or using a Web search engine. At the end of the session, students were asked to rate their success in finding answers based upon the chosen sources. This format worked well for three years, but with the higher level of computer competency, Web savvy, and database searching familiarity in each succeeding freshman class, training needs changed accordingly. Starting in the fall 2003 semester, the training program places greater emphasis on the small-group learning experience by integrating the database and electronic resources instruction into that forum.

EVALUATION METHODS

Since 1999, evaluations of each training session have been conducted online. LXR, a testing software program, had been adopted to administer quizzes in the first year of the curriculum. By answering the evaluation questions online, the students became comfortable with the mechanics of using the LXR software (such as finding out where it was located on the desktop, signing in, logging off, etc.), relieving them of "technological anxiety" when it came time to take a graded quiz.

Evaluation of the training program is accomplished with a seven-question survey as students complete each training session. The results are compiled and analyzed by the training group. The Office of Medical Education surveys each class at least once a year. Questions are designed to elicit information about how comfortable students are using technology, which programs are used the most, and how technology is being applied within the curriculum. The analysis of these survey results will help identify areas that might need more emphasis in the future.

CONCLUSION

Looking back on the development of the ThinkPad project, a pattern of action, reaction, and adaptation emerges. One of the keys to the success of the WFUSM approach has been willingness to change instruction delivery based on experience and student feedback. The training workgroup has been responsive to the evaluations gathered from every session and has tried to incorporate suggested changes into the next cycle. From the very first year, the training program has been successful because it delivered an extensive program of training to the smallest class size possible in the shortest amount of time. The concept of conducting initial laptop training in the same room where students use laptops during the curriculum day helped make the training coherent and logical to the new student. Another successful element was the consistency with which the training material was delivered. The training script has reduced the amount of time needed to "train the trainer" as well as ensuring uniformity in the information being delivered. Willing and able volunteers among the student body and library and Academic Computing staff also contributed to the success of the program by undertaking the computer distribution training.

The library has worked closely with Academic Computing, Medical Education, and individual faculty and students to create a dynamic educational technology and information resources program that has been very successful in achieving the original information management goals set out by the Educational Computing Committee in 1996. In the process of planning and teaching the original Mobile Computing Project, Coy C. Carpenter Library is regarded by others within the WFUSM community as a legitimate participant in future technological training programs.

APPENDIX A:
THINKPAD EXERCISES AND ANSWERS

Exercises

Exercise 1: Go to the mouse settings and make certain the trailing feature on your cursor is "on."

Exercise 2: Create a shortcut to Windows Explorer.

Exercise 3: Create a shortcut to Microsoft Word.

Exercise 4: Create a shortcut to *Stedman's Medical Dictionary* (hint: file name is Scmd10).

Exercise 5: Arrange the icons by type; rearrange icons using autoarrange.

Exercise 6: Delete the shortcut titled "How to Connect to the Network Printer."

Exercise 7: Go to Microsoft Word. Reduce the opened window to a button on the taskbar. Reopen Microsoft Word from the taskbar. Maximize the screen and then exit the application.

Exercise 8: Add the calculator to your Start menu. Remove the calculator from your Start menu.

Exercise 9: Create a folder; title it "Papers written first semester 1997."

Exercise 10: Delete the folder you created titled "Papers written first semester 1997."

Exercise 11: Create a folder "ScreenCam" in the My Documents folder, *then* copy "startup.scm" from the A:\ drive to folder "ScreenCam."

Exercise 12: Open ScreenCam player and play "startup.scm."

Answers to Exercises

Exercise 1:
1. Choose Start-Settings-Control Panel, then double-click the mouse icon.
2. Choose motion tab.
3. Choose pointer trail.

Exercise 2:
1. Choose Start-Find-Files or Folders.
2. Type "Windows Explorer" in box. Click on Find Now.
3. Click on Explorer and drag to desktop.
4. Close the window.

Exercise 3:
1. Choose Start-Find-Files or Folders.
2. Type "Microsoft Word" in the box. Click on Find Now.
3. Click on Word shortcut and drag to the desktop.
4. Close the window.

Exercise 4:
1. Right click on blank portion of the desktop.
2. Choose New.
3. Click on Shortcut.
4. Click on Browse.
5. Double-click on Program Files.
6. Double-click on Scmd10.
7. Click on Scmdwin.
8. Click on Open.
9. Click on Next.
10. Select a name (suggestion: "Stedman's").
11. Click Finish.

Exercise 5:
1. Right click on desktop.
2. Choose Arrange Icons.
3. From flyaway menu, click on Auto Arrange.
4. Right click on desktop.
5. Choose Arrange Icons.
6. Click on Arrange by Type.
7. Move icons into two groups.
8. Right click on desktop.
9. Choose Arrange Icons.
10. From flyaway menu, click on Auto Arrange.

Exercise 6:
1. Right click on icon.
2. Choose Delete.
3. Choose Yes.

Exercise 7:
1. Click on Microsoft Word icon from the desktop.
2. Click on the minimize button.
3. Click on Microsoft Word from the taskbar.
4. Click on the close button.

Exercise 8:
1. Choose Start-Settings-Taskbar.
2. Click on Start menu programs.
3. Click on Add.
4. Click on Browse.
5. Open Windows folder for calculator.
6. Choose calculator by double clicking.
7. Choose Next.
8. Choose Start menu folder. Click on Next.
9. Change the name if desired. Click on Finish. Click on OK. Part 2 of exercise is basically the same except click on Remove.

Exercise 9:
1. Choose My Documents from the desktop.
2. Right click. Choose New.
3. Choose Folder.
4. Name folder "Papers written first semester 1997."

Exercise 10:
1. Choose My Documents from the desktop.
2. Right click on the folder to be deleted.
3. Click Delete.
4. Click Yes.

Exercise 11:
1. Choose My Documents from the desktop.
2. Right click. Choose New.
3. Choose Folder.
4. Name folder "ScreenCam."
5. Double-click My Computer icon on desktop.
6. Double-click A:\.
7. Click on "startup.scm" to highlight.
8. Choose Edit, then Copy.
9. Double-click ScreenCam folder in My Documents window.
10. Choose Edit, then Paste.
11. Close all open windows.

Exercise 12:
1. Choose Start-Programs-Accessories-Lotus Applications-ScreenCam Player.
2. Click on Open File.
3. Click folder or click arrow.
4. Choose Userdata, then choose ScreenCam folder.
5. Click on File name.
6. Click Open.
7. Click Play.

APPENDIX B: THINKPAD TRAINING EVALUATION SURVEY

Please take a few minutes to answer these questions about the training session you just completed.

1. How would you rate the clarity of presentation of this training session?
   a. Very unclear
   b. Somewhat unclear
   c. Clear
   d. Very clear
2. How useful were the handout materials (if any) for this training session?
   a. Not useful at all
   b. Minimally useful
   c. Moderately useful
   d. Very useful
   e. There were no handouts
3. The amount of content presented in this training session was
   a. Much less than I would have liked
   b. A little less than I would have liked
   c. About right
   d. A little more than I would have liked
   e. A lot more than I would have liked
4. Given your previous experience, how appropriate was the level of training for you?
   a. Much too difficult
   b. A little too difficult
   c. About right
   d. A little too easy
   e. Much too easy
5. How useful do you believe this training course was in preparing you to use the skills it covered?
   a. Not useful at all
   b. Minimally useful
   c. Moderately useful
   d. Very useful
6. What did you find *most* useful about this training session?
7. What did you find *least* useful about this training session?
8. If you have additional comments or suggestions, please add them here:

Index

Page numbers followed by the letter "f" indicate figures; those followed by the letter "i" indicate illustrations; and those followed by the letter "t" indicate tables.